Awakening Through Sleep

MAR DE CARLO is an international entrepreneur motivational speaker, holistic curriculum developer, educator, author, health, life & business coach, artist and mother.

She has completed a multitude of certification programs, workshops, classes, and trainings over the last twenty-five years. Throughout this time, she has coached, managed, mentored, trained and advised thousands of professionals and businesses worldwide.

She is a gifted intuitive who has pioneered several new conceptual cutting-edge holistic programs in the parenting and health fields. She is known for her creative, unconventional and integrative approach that bridges a variety of systems that has transformed thousands of lives throughout fifty-nine countries.

She is the founder of:

- International Parenting & Health Institute
- Association of Professional Sleep Consultants
- International Academy of Baby Planner Professionals
- Business Sanctuary
- Physical Awakening

Awakening Through Sleep

A transformational and spiritual guide for pregnancy, adult and child sleep

MAR DE CARLO

Awakening Through Sleep

The information contained herein reflects only the opinion of the author. In no way is it to be considered medical or product advice. Specific medical advice should be obtained from a licensed health care practitioner. Consult with your doctor before you begin any sleep, fitness, exercise, nutrition, diet, weight loss, heart attack or stroke risk reduction program or other change in health and lifestyle. This information is in no way meant to treat, cure or prevent any trauma, disease or illness from happening.

The author has provided this book and the information on it for consumer education purposes only. The author is not engaged in rendering professional advice or services to the individual reader. Therefore, you should consult with your personal physician or other health-care professional if you have any healthcare or therapy related questions or before embarking on a health, fitness or lifestyle program. If a medical problem appears or persists, do not disregard or delay seeking medical advice from your personal physician or other qualified healthcare provider based on something you read in the book. Accordingly, the author, expressly disclaims any liability, loss, damage, or injury caused by information contained in this book.

Mention of specific companies, organizations, or authorities in this book does not imply endorsement by the author or publisher, nor does mention of specific companies, organizations, or authorities imply their endorsement of this book, its author, or the publisher.

The author has strived to be as accurate and complete as possible in the creation of this book, notwithstanding the fact that she does not warrant or represent at any time that the contents within are accurate due to the rapidly changing nature of the internet. The author does not assume any responsibility for errors or changes that occur after publication.

Internet addresses were accurate at the time this book went to press. Library of Congress Cataloging-in-Publication has been applied for.

ISBN 978-0-578-43396-7

Cover Emily Genevish

Editor Shanen Ilg

Contents

Introduction

After giving birth, sleep can be a great challenge for the entire household: not just a child issue but a family issue. When a child is experiencing sleep challenges, the whole family is affected. Often, these families have been sleep-deprived for weeks and sometimes months, which can have negative and traumatic effects even after experiencing a healthy and powerful birth.

How we address this issue as professionals and parents can lead us down a path of ease or frustration. Infant and child sleep carries with it not only so much controversy, but also in many cases causes overwhelm, stress and a disruption of the family connection.

When an infant is experiencing sleep problems, families seek many resources for support from their doctors, friends, forums, books and child sleep consultants. Routinely such consultants are hired a few months after the baby is born, and typically they resort to behavioral methods known as sleep training. There are many methods of sleep training which commonly fall under three main categories: *cry it out, no cry* or *gentle sleep.*

While these approaches can be helpful and provide some relief and solutions, generally they do not address the root cause. As a result, they often overlook many important factors including parents' own behavior, sleep habits, lifestyle, beliefs, expectations, and how these influence and play a critical role in their child's sleep.

Sleep training methods more often than not, do not leave room for customization and make assumptions about child sleep challenges. They customarily do not consider a thorough investigative process assessing a whole family's lifestyle, health and history and often do not acknowledge one of the most important tools for parenting: intuition.

Anti and pro-sleep foods, emotional wellbeing, parent's behavior, self-care, temperaments, expectations and attitudes are a few more examples of influences and factors also frequently overlooked in typical behavioral approaches. There is now the recognition that such approaches can be very confusing because they commonly do not consider the *context* of the child's sleep issues and the infant's natural inbuilt sleep tendencies. Unless the context and natural mechanisms are considered, there's the chance that "therapies" will be spurious and even unhelpful. The goal is to improve a child's sleep quality, the wellbeing of the whole family unit, not just – or even --to keep the house quiet at night.

It also important to recognize that while we sleep, our brains never do. They are constantly working, even during sleep -- especially during sleep. The critical role of sleep to overall health and function has into focus much more in the last few years. Previously thought of as merely rest, it now is clear that sleep has some very critical functions.

The first is the consolidation of experiences into memories and neural pathways. This is essential for learning. And one of the misconceptions about infant sleep is that because a baby does not appear to demonstrate much cognitive function, the consolidation of memories and cognitive function at this stage is not important. Nothing could be further from the truth! A newborn child's brain is developing at amazing speed and one might even conclude that quality sleep is more critical for brain development in infancy than it is during the later stages of life. Babies are laying the neural foundations for all their behaviors and experiences.

The second critical function of sleep is the clearing of nerve cell toxic waste. In later years, poor sleep is associated with the buildup of tau protein and amyloid, which are highly associated with dementia. While poor waste removal from a baby's brain might not lead to such immediate problems, it surely interferes with brain development.

In addition, sleep training methods can be very limiting as most behavioral approaches do not acknowledge the important biological need and influence of secure attachment in human development. Another interesting consideration is that sleep training methods do not address sleep during pregnancy. When I first became familiarized with the child sleep consulting industry and profession, I was very surprised that the support and education for child sleep began at four, five and six months after birth and not earlier. There is a great opportunity during pregnancy, not only to support mom and baby but also take preventative measures to minimize future problems.

When we look at the statistics of, for example, sleep during pregnancy, the percentage of pregnant women experiencing sleep challenges is very high. According to the National Sleep Foundation, 78% of pregnant women experience disturbed sleep. But as high as this statistic is, the perception, norm and the cultural standard is that having disturbed sleep during pregnancy is part of a normal process and we should just accept it.

Since there is very little support and education to address sleep challenges during pregnancy and for newborns, I felt deeply moved to do something about it. There are many preventative measures that can be taken to minimize future problems and create healthy lifestyle habits. I became the first in the child sleep consultant industry to develop and launch my Holistic Adult and Child Sleep Certification program in 2012 that trains professionals to begin supporting families with sleep education during pregnancy. My program and approach have been well-received in 46 countries and are currently represented in 10 languages.

I acknowledge how much sleep training methods have supported and saved so many families. Every family is doing the best they can by using what works for them. I am not suggesting sleep training methods are bad or families who have used them have done something wrong. If it worked for you, great! I understand sleep training method developers are very well intentioned and supportive. But with all this being shared, I have found the perspective and approach used to solve child sleep challenges via behavioral methods to be limiting and disempowering in so many ways. I have witnessed many families who resorted to sleep training because they were unaware of vital factors influencing sleep. I have also witnessed many families who have not uncovered the root of their child's sleep challenge and resorting to sleep training only made matters worse. Many families feel like failures and have held guilt, frustration and stress because they were fed limiting and misleading perspectives about child sleep development through sleep training. My intention is not to convince anyone to not use sleep training. If you feel firmly called to using it, that is your prerogative and choice. I completely honor that you know what the best course of action is for you and your family to resolve your child's sleep.

The information and insights I share in my book are intended as an opportunity to expand and deepen your learning and understanding of sleep with an empowering and life-changing perspective for those with whom it resonates. It also is intended to invite and motivate you to acknowledge and awaken to the intelligence of your inner guide and power held within your body so that you develop a keen sense of awareness that will guide you and your child toward optimal well-being.

As a result of all these considerations, I have become deeply passionate about pregnancy, adult and child sleep. In 2014, I began my journey to share my vision and expanded perspective in the form of a book which has continuously evolved through my research, experience, studies and meditation.

Throughout my life, I have considered myself a skeptic. When faced with a challenge, before I assume and draw conclusions, I investigate, research, reflect, make connections, use logic, experience, experimentation, evaluation and then invite meditation, feeling and intuition to digest, integrate and guide me toward the most optimal solution. In this same fashion, I teach my clients and professionals I train to do the same.

I feel grateful for the opportunity to share what I have learned with all of you. All my research, findings and insights are available for you today because of my commitment to my personal and professional development. I have been blessed with the opportunity to do the inner work and meditation, as well as study, train, and practice in each area of the wheel of health and life. A variety of gurus, experts, colleagues and clients from all walks of life have contributed to my development and education in psychology, neuroscience, nutrition, anatomy and physiology, exercise, sleep, dance, child development, human development, spirituality, yoga, pilates, stress management, pregnancy, birth, parenting, meditation, conflict resolution and much more.

Some people see a glass half-empty; some people see a glass half-full; some people see a glass with water in it and some people see a hard object containing a soft object. Some people like myself, see all of these elements combined, connecting and understanding the relationship and impact between them. Similarly, my book presents a combined elements approach that welcomes an integrative and holistic perspective of pregnancy, child and adult sleep.

As a result, I am not going to spend time covering or extensively reviewing sleep science and sleep training, because there are plenty of books out there that already do so.

Rather I, present and share information on the many influences of sleep that you most often will not find covered or spoken about in your average book, magazine article or mainstream sleep consultation.

My perspectives may challenge your beliefs about sleep, provide you deeper insight and an opportunity to resolve your or your child's sleep challenges with room to support your own well-being and strengthen your family connection.

This information may not only help you uncover the root of your or your child's sleep challenges but may also transform and expand your and your child's life.

I titled my book "Awakening Through Sleep" because I have not only discovered sleep to be a key factor to maintain optimal health of one's physical body, but also for human development, providing us an opportunity to awaken to greater insight, creativity, expansion and evolution of one's mind, intuition and spirit.

Osho, an Indian spiritual leader, teacher and mystic, once gave a talk titled "The Inner Journey" in 1968 on Right Sleep that I resonate with deeply and matches my experience and findings.

He says,

> *The thing which has been harmed the most in the development of human civilization is sleep. From the day man discovered artificial light, his sleep has become very troubled. And as more and more gadgets started falling into man's hands, he started feeling that sleep is an unnecessary thing, too much time is wasted in it. The time when we are asleep is a complete waste. So, the less sleep we can do with the better. It does not occur to people that sleep has any kind of contribution to the deeper processes of life. They think that the time spent sleeping is time gone to waste, so the less they sleep the better; the more quickly they reduce the amount of sleep, the better.*

We have not even noticed that the cause behind all the illnesses, all the disorders that have entered man's life is lack of sleep. The person who cannot sleep rightly cannot live rightly.

Sleep is not a waste of time. The eight hours of sleep are not being wasted; rather, because of those eight hours, you are able to stay awake for sixteen hours. Otherwise, you would not be able to stay awake all that time.

During those eight hours life-energy is accumulated, your life gets revitalized, the centers of your brain and heart calm down and your life functions from your navel center. For those eight hours of sleep, you have again become one with nature and with existence. That is why you become revitalized.

Sleep needs to come back into man's life. Really, there is no alternative, no other step, for the psychological health of humanity than that sleep should be made compulsory by law for the next one or two hundred years.

It is very important for a meditator to see to it that he sleeps properly and enough. And one more thing needs to be understood – right sleep will be different for everybody. It will not be equal because the body has needs which are different for everyone...according to age and to many other elements.

Thank you for taking the time to open yourself up to another way of perceiving, understanding, and approaching pregnancy, adult and child sleep.

In order to prepare ourselves for this reading journey, let's explore my *Physical Awakening* method in the following chapter.

Mar De Carlo

Physical Awakening

Physical Awakening Method

"You should sit in meditation for 20 minutes every day, unless you're too busy. Then you should sit for an hour."
Zen Proverb

Most of us have not taken the time to invest in our wellbeing. Quite often when we're on the go, we have so many things to do and errands to run. It feels almost impossible to believe that taking a step back can help us go forward more. Therefore, we are running around with a partially working physical machine that struggles to feel well rested and at peace.

Taking a pause and allowing ourselves to reflect, meditate, connect, activate and integrate optimizes our well-being. It allows us to get a lot more done. It brings clarity, focus and ease, enhancing our quality of life. More importantly, we begin to awaken to ourselves.

Sadhguru Jaggi Vasudev, author of Inner Engineer says,

> *Just about everything today comes with a user's manual, whether it is in the box or is an internet*

link. Sometimes these manuals are wordy and complicated or only contain confusing pictures but they still represent a resource that hopefully enables the product to function properly. They provide some guidelines that allow us to know the ins and outs of the product.

But what about a human being? Have you ever heard a parent declare "I need a user's manual!" Countless authors have supplied an abundance of advice for parents and others. The problem is most of the advice is conflicting.

So how much do you know about your own life? How much do you understand the workings of your body, mind, and emotions?

The body is a supercomputer that has been given to us. It can't be found in any bookstore. However, if you pay enough attention to the fundamental life that you are, everything you want to know about life can be found right here. Spirituality means start reading the user's manual.

Because many of us believe we are limited on time, we deprive ourselves of being present and fully connecting with the intelligence of our bodies. When it comes to reflecting and learning, we often do not fully grasp or absorb real knowledge, just bits and pieces. We are not fully engaged or present because our mind is filled with so many other thoughts and distractions. Therefore, our user's manual is not clear.

I developed a Physical Awakening Method, my personal meditation variation, after giving birth to my company, Physical Awakening in 2005.

I consider a "physical awakening" to occur when one's body, mind and spirit fully activate, integrate and function optimally as whole. As a result, one feels most alive, present and can function at one's ultimate best. One's mind becomes organized and one's intuitive muscle is also strengthened. This is consciousness, the ultimate intelligence.

"It is through your body that you realize you are a spark of divinity." ~B.K.S. Iyengar

I have experienced many "physical awakenings" when prioritizing my well-being. Many of my "physical awakenings" were born from moments when I was deeply present, physically connected, well-rested, nourished and relaxed. During these moments I was gifted with profound insights, creativity, inspiration, clarity and wellbeing that led to a deeper understanding and connection with myself.

Although used daily, I particularly love to use this method when I'm learning or receiving guidance. Usually, when we're learning or reading, without being conscious of it, we are disconnected from our body and stuck in limiting beliefs and identities. Another factor is that my mind can become so absorbed, that I have experienced headaches after a reading or learning experience. If I'm in a workshop that's three or four days, for example, and we're going four or five hours at a time or longer, it is not unusual for me to experience a headache because of how hard my mind has been processing and absorbing information.

As a result, I began integrating a "physical awakening" experience with my body to support my mind and spirit, making the learning experience much more enjoyable and effective.

I invite you to experiment, explore, reflect, and take some time and space to digest what is shared- not just with your mind, but also with the presence of your body to get the most out of my book.

Give yourself an opportunity to take some space, feel your body, feel your breath as you read. Why? Because when your mind and body are present, connected and focused, aka, "physically awake", you are giving yourself a chance to learn in the most optimal way that is appropriate for you.

When we have an opportunity to learn optimally, we can expand our way of thinking, and develop and evolve in a way that feels most alive and functional.

The key to enhanced awareness is a state of complete relaxation and stillness, where energy can be free to flow through you without distraction. Any tension will distract your brain from full attention.

Before we get into the relaxation of your body and stillness of your mind, explore moving your body for a few minutes. This can be a movement that feels good to your body, especially an activity that you enjoy. For example: Tai Chi, Yoga, dance, gentle stretching.

Moving your body is associated with an increase in chemicals are in charge of focus and learning, like BDNF, Brain-Derived Neurotropic Factor. Physical activity just prior to learning has been shown to maximize it in some incredible ways.

Once you have moved in a way that you find enjoyable and fun for about five to ten minutes, it's time to relax the body and still the mind:

Find a place, devoid of distractions.

Sit in a comfortable position.

Close your eyes and connect within.

Since so much of our sensory input is connecting outside or taking the outside in, connecting within allows you to feel yourself from the inside out.

Keeping your mouth closed, breath normally in and out of your nose.

Begin to feel your breath.

Without trying to fix or change anything, notice your inhalation as your breath comes in and travels through your body. Do this for a few breaths.

After a few breaths, feel your inhalation moving through your nose, into your skull, into you're your neck, into your chest and then expanding into your belly.

Then begin to feel your exhalation leaving your body, as your belly flattens, your chest softens, and your breath releases out through your nose.

Using your sense of awareness and intuition to guide you. If you want to take your experience deeper, after a few rounds, you can begin bringing awareness to the quality of your breath: how long you inhale and exhale, noticing if your breath is quick or slow and then continuing to lengthen and slow down your breath.

Next, allow your breath to remain as you have just been practicing and begin to scan your body starting from your feet to your head or from your head to your feet.

Choose an upright posture that you know is going to keep you comfortable but alert. Position your posture in a way that easily allows you to scan each area of your body.

For example, sitting in a chair or on a meditation cushion, or kneeling on a meditation cushion or chair.

Starting from the crown of your head or from the base of your feet, visit each part of your body:

Become aware of a body part like the crown of your head, for example. Feel the crown of your head, connect with it and feel it activate by imagining you are turning on a light switch. Then take one full inhalation and exhalation while remaining present with the crown of your head. If you feel any tension, pause. Take a deeper slower breath in and slowly release the tension out. If pausing and taking a deeper, slower breath does not release tension, feel free to take a moment to move the appropriate body part, for example, shoulders, so that the tension disappears.

Next, move on to another part of your body. Repeat the steps and keep doing this until you have visited each area of your body feeling each part fully activated and present.

For a deeper experience, take the time to scan not just the larger body parts, but the smaller ones. For example, your nose, mouth, ears, fingers, toes, nails, etc........

Once you have completed scanning and activating each area of your body, notice how you feel. If you feel more active, present and relaxed, you are ready to integrate your present state with your reading and learning experience. You are ready to expand your awareness.

Holistic Science of Sleep Method

The word "science" is derived from the Latin word *scientia*, which is knowledge based on demonstrable and reproducible data, according to the Merriam-Webster Dictionary.

According to the Oxford Dictionary, "science" is the intellectual and practical activity encompassing the systematic study of the structure and behavior of the physical and natural world through observation and experimentation.

True to these definitions, science aims for measurable results through testing and analysis. Science is based on fact, not opinion or preferences. However, science is not free from bias – it's a human activity after all.

Behavioral research is prone to misinterpretations and at best can only show an association between variables, which may or may not be causal.

When conducting research, scientists use the "Scientific Method" to collect measurable, empirical evidence in an experiment related to a hypothesis.

Of course, we can always gather much more reliable information on each situation than can be captured in major research. And, of course, we measure outcomes.

Generalizations and assumptions are often made about sleep. However, the sleep challenge we or our child experiences is individual and unique. While our own or our child's sleep challenge may seem to share similar traits to a sleep challenge someone else is experiencing, we still need to approach the issue with a thorough investigative process, keen sense of awareness and open curiosity.

Therefore, I developed and termed my approach as the "Holistic Science of Sleep Method", an adult and child sleep approach that integrates holistic thinking with the scientific method to provide conscious and optimal solutions to adult and child sleep challenges.

My Holistic Science of Sleep Method investigates, evaluates and uncovers the root of sleep challenges leading one to properly address imbalances in human function that may be impacting sleep and leading to adult and child sleep challenges.

In other words, we are looking at the whole, not just the parts, and integrating those two worlds together. Many sleep experts do not do this. They just look at the parts and don't integrate them in order to see the whole picture which is necessary for a comprehensive solution. Or they see similar symptoms and will advise a one-size-fits-all solution.

As I stated in my introductory chapter, when an adult, pregnant woman or parents of a child experience a sleep challenge, one of the most common paths they take to solve the "problem" is one of public inquisition, usually with the general questions being asked right from the start.

Quite often, one may seek the support of online forums, books, doctors, friends or public groups where the root of sleep issues is not being addressed. Rather general questions are asked, and general answers are given based on the others' experiences, limited training or paradigm, which rarely is holistic in nature.

Most questions asked do not include important details about their lifestyle or physical and emotional health history that need to be factored in before receiving basic advice or suggestions. There are so many forces that affect sleep. In order to get to the root of the challenge we must first investigate the strongest forces that affect sleep in order to first rule those "causes" out.

Anyone who is answering health or sleep questions while knowing little to nothing about the client's health history, blood work, diet, emotional wellbeing and all the rest of it, is just throwing darts at best, hoping to knock out the main "problem". Rarely is there just one main "problem" or factor; more often than not there are many forces acting upon a family preventing them from getting good sleep.

For example, one of my graduates shared with me that a mother of a 3.5-month-old baby who reached out to a sleep consultant from another school, was told to do *cry it out* at 3.5 months, although the consultant informed her that it might not work until the 4-month mark because her baby might be developmentally not ready yet.

This sleep consultant who advised *cry it out* had not checked any of the foundations that my graduate holistically trained to investigate. The mother of this baby has serious breastfeeding issues and her baby is also allergic to cow's milk protein. The mother found out all this information when she started working together with my graduate. Her emotional well-being and self-care, as well as her husband's emotional well-being was never considered with the prior consultant who advised her to just do *cry it out*. Basic sleep environment issues like noise from the neighbors or blue/white light in the bedroom were also never mentioned as possible sleep disruptors. The underlying medical causes and basic sleep environment factors were not taken into consideration with this family until my graduate became involved and applied my Holistic Science of Sleep Method.

One important part of my work involves teaching my clients and students to understand the many factors that regulate and influence sleep through the various stages of human development. Another important part of my work involves evaluating parents' physical and emotional well-being to ensure appropriate measures are taken to support their health. Parents commonly forget to care for themselves and as a result leave barely any room to have the energy to care for another. One more important part of my work is teaching my clients and students to be open to learning from a child. Often parents and professionals rely so heavily and get hyper focused on books and rigid methods that they overlook the most important source of information, their child. A child is also like a book that is providing us essential information from which we can learn. Children teach and guide us just as much as we do them. We just have to be willing to be open and tune in.

My Holistic Science of Sleep Method provides the framework and understanding that supports adults, pregnant women, parents and professionals in learning, addressing and resolving the many factors creating a sleep challenge, in order of importance.

A Holistic Science of Sleep Method practitioner understands and honors that our children's bodies do not need to technically be "trained" to sleep. By nature's design, human bodies are already developmentally programmed to sleep and will do so if we support the process.

A Holistic Science of Sleep Method practitioner will empower each of their clients to understand the function and mechanics of sleep and how it relates to health and lifestyle while helping their clients develop a keen sense of awareness and strong relationship with their body.

A Holistic Science of Sleep Method practitioner will address and analyze internal and external forces individually, hitting upon the major (and often overlooked) factors early on in the process. But in order to do this, a great amount of detail and information needs to be collected and evaluated with regard to their client's health, emotional well-being and lifestyle history, including their recent blood tests from their last doctor's visit.

A Holistic Science of Sleep Method practitioner may need to refer their clients to the right health practitioners who can rule out and analyze certain imbalances. There is rarely just one problem affecting someone's sleep. It is usually a combination of many factors/forces, each one building upon the other. Therefore, a holistic approach is suitable.

Most importantly, a Holistic Science of Sleep Method practitioner will guide their clients to a lifestyle that supports optimal sleep for themselves and their whole family.

Foundational Factors

Below are some examples of foundational factors and solutions my Holistic Science of Sleep Method investigates, assesses, addresses and uncovers:

- o Medical issues to be ruled out or referred out

- o Adult and child's physical and emotional states and needs

- o Sleep history, birth history and health history of both adult and child

- o Quality and breathing pattern of both child and adult

- o Stress levels, energy, rhythms, temperaments of adult and child

- Quality of relationships, alignments, connections and support systems

- Physical bedroom and home environment

- Sleep and wake times, food and drink intake and activity level in a 24-hour period and consistent basis

- Recent medical visits, medications, and any diagnoses to assess physical health

- Full blood panel, that is evaluated by their doctor, checking for any chemical imbalances or vitamin deficiencies (for example, iron, magnesium and vitamin D deficiencies may inhibit sleep)

- Possible food and other sensitivities/intolerances/allergies diagnosed by a highly qualified holistic naturopath who can provide various testing options from elimination diet to blood work o Adults' beliefs, expectations, and behavior regarding their child's sleep and their own sleep

As you can see, almost anything can interfere with a child's or adult's ability to sleep. When a human being encounters a new biological or chemical substance, their system will be challenged to defend itself. Obviously young infants are more vulnerable to such influences as they are encountering many things for the first time.

What may seem harmless to you, like a new deodorant, perfume or air freshener, can be a novel challenge to an infant.

A vaccine may have general utility, but everyone will respond differently based on immune system function.

New supplements, foods and medicines also have an individualized biological impact that certainly can affect the many complex interactions necessary for restorative sleep.

Interactions with new pets (yours or somebody else's) or even a visit to a petting zoo can create reactions that disturb your child's internal environment.

So, it is important to tune in and assess any influences on your child's body that could be responsible for changes in sleep.

In addition to these assessments, it is critical that one has the right mindset and tools to interpret the results and implement effective action:

Mindset Examples

o Understanding the language of crying

o Reframing limiting labels, terms and perspectives

o Reprograming expectations, attitudes and beliefs about sleep

o Considering sleep as a social and shared experience under one roof and not a solitary one o Considering sleep as a family sleep issue and not just a child sleep issue

o Working with a team-led approach versus a parent-led or baby-led approach

o Embracing sleep challenges as an opportunity to expand, grow and improve one's own and family's well-being.

Practical Tools

There are many practical and realistic tools and techniques to support optimal sleep for a family. These may include but not limited to:

o Inviting and creating a support system

o Strengthening relationships between family members and connection with self

o Developing a keen sense of awareness and strong connection to your body

o Meditating

- o Being the change: Understanding your sleep history and modeling healthy sleep for your child
- o Supporting your child to play and be fully expressed throughout the day

- o Establishing a bedtime ritual and routine

- o Honoring gradual transitions and supporting any change your child is experiencing

- o Integrating relaxation as part of your and your family's lifestyle

- o Taking daily pauses: training your body to release tension throughout the day by taking short pauses for breathing and meditation exercises

- o Eating a pro-sleep, anti-inflammatory diet

- o Staying well-hydrated

o   Physical activity on a regular basis

o   Ensuring bedroom environment is "green" and creating a sleep sanctuary (check indoor air quality, electronics are shut off)

o   Getting sunshine upon waking

o   Following a regular schedule throughout the day and allowing for transitions between day and nigh

o   Trusting that your child knows how to sleep and wants to sleep

o   Being open to learning from your child how to sleep

o   Focusing on your progress and celebrating your success

This latter point is very important and is often one of the fallacies and failures of sleep interventions. Now that we have covered the basics of foundational factors, mindset examples and practical tools, let's explore these concepts in greater detail.

Reframing
Labels, Thoughts, Beliefs & Perspectives
about Sleep

It might seem that labels help us to figure out people and their challenges a lot easier, but I have found that quite often labels lead to quick assumptions that divide us from one another and overlook many important factors and lessons.

"Labels are for filing. Labels are for clothing. Labels are not for people." ~ Martina Navratilova

Labels

Some common examples of how parenting styles are defined:

o   Attachment Parenting
o   Helicopter Parenting
o   Authoritative Parenting
o   Permissive Parenting
o   Tiger Parenting

Some common examples of how children are defined by their parents or caregivers when not sleeping well:

o   Bad-Tempered
o   Hyper
o   Manipulative

- ○ Challenging
- ○ Resistant

Some common examples of how adults define themselves with sleep:

- ○ Night Owl
- ○ Insomniac
- ○ Light Sleeper
- ○ Deep Sleeper
- ○ Bad Sleeper
- ○ Good Sleeper

"Labels obscure the beauty that lies beneath them. With just one word, we can suck the life out of anything - even an entire species. Labels kill our curiosity about them, prevent us from exploring" .... (and growing). ~ John Ptacek

Often, I'm asked if my child sleep approach is attachment parenting or sleep training based on cry it out, gentle or no-cry approaches. My response is that my approach is not based on a behavioral method or parenting style but rather it is based on understanding the internal or external factors surrounding physical, mental, emotional health, lifestyle, relationships and environment that influence the quality and function of sleep. The same goes for my approach to adult sleep.

Question Your Thoughts and Beliefs

"Do you belong to your thoughts or do your thoughts belong to you?" ~ Sadhguru

"Don't believe everything you think." ~Robert Fulghum

When it comes to pregnancy, adult and child sleep, there are many beliefs and misconceptions about sleep and the right way to sleep.

Sleep can be seen as a huge problem or enemy. Some don't like sleep or wish sleep never existed. For example, "Oh, I've got to sleep but I have things to get done." It's like, if they could go without sleep, they would, but they do not prioritize it. That's part of the problem; we live in a society where the important function of rest and sleep for optimal health and personal development is greatly misunderstood and undervalued. There are many misconceptions and limiting beliefs about sleep. The more you do and the more you can take on, the stronger you appear to be, right? The more of a superhuman you appear to be. But when we think this way, we go against our own nature and as a result, pay a price.

Where do these beliefs come from?

Before we answer this question, let's look at the distinction between narratives and beliefs.

In order to expand our thinking, it's important to identify our beliefs. That way, we can look at whether or not they are true, and why we have them.

Narratives are stories or ideas and supposed "facts" that you have heard or generated and simply accepted. You haven't investigated them deeply and don't have much emotional connection to them. For example, you might have heard or read that all infants must sleep 16 hours a day, and just assumed this was an accurate statement.

A belief has much more emotional power. You are committed to the belief and really own it. This might take the form of something like, "My baby should learn to behave and sleep through the night."

Narratives are easier to give up than beliefs. Beliefs, on the other hand, are hard to put aside. However, when you take a moment to question your beliefs and understand where they came from, you can learn new perspectives, have "facts" clarified and integrate them into your understanding.

Uncovering Our Beliefs

We draw our beliefs from so many places. They are very much influenced by a whole host of factors.
Understanding those influences on a deep level provides us an opportunity to really explore our beliefs, re-evaluate them and decide whether they are truly serving us or not.

Our beliefs can be generated from observations, personal experience, science, authority, assumptions, facts, law, policies, emotions, subconscious and so on.

Some of the greatest influences on our beliefs come from ancestors, parents, friends, teachers, religions, experiences, cultural, traditions, television, movies, schools, books, magazines, radio shows, experts and doctors. What is important is to recognize the context in which all these sources generated the beliefs in question. For example, many religious nutritional beliefs stem from times when there was no refrigeration. The proscriptions and combinations of foods were realistically based on avoiding potential health risks. That context doesn't apply today but, did centuries ago.

In order to be open to our beliefs, we must be curious enough to question and examine them. This will transform our beliefs, especially the ones we find that are limiting and not serving us. But first we need to understand whether these beliefs are really ours, or have we merely taken on someone else's?

For example, is it my belief that babies manipulate or is that someone else's idea? What is my belief based on? Is it based on my experiences as a child? Is it based on an authority and what they say? Is it based on emotion, intuition, logic, or science? Where is this belief coming from? Is it true? How long has this belief been with me? What is the earliest memory of having this belief? How did it feel to have this belief? Is it really serving me and everyone around me? Does this belief support me?

The key to getting at the root of any challenge is to understand our beliefs. When we examine where they are coming from and how they are serving (or not serving) us, we have the potential to discover a solution and evolve. In order for this to happen, we must be fully conscious of our beliefs.

We're going to begin by looking at core beliefs. There are many ways and techniques of locating, identifying and understanding what core beliefs are. Some examples include analysis, journaling and observing your thoughts and emotions.

Sometimes it's just pure observation: "Hmm, what am I saying and thinking? What do I find myself really strongly feeling about?" You can begin by asking some top-level questions like: What beliefs are you aware of? What voices do you hear and what do they say? What do you want to change and why? What do you want to create that you're unable to? What's interfering with your life? What is the belief that underpins or supports the situation?

What is it that is making you so angry? What do you think is unfair and what are you afraid of? When did you first have this belief?

I find meditation, in particular Vipassana meditation, to be very helpful in slowing my mind and identifying my core beliefs. Find a technique that works best for you and put it into practice. If you choose one that doesn't work, choose another.

For us to maintain the illusion of consistency, human beings resort to several cognitive biases. One of these is the *confirmational bias* in which we seek out evidence that supports our beliefs and ignore the evidence that doesn't. This way we can avoid the problem of constantly dealing with our inconsistent views.

There are other biases, including the *Halo Effect* coined by psychologist Edward Thorndike. In this bias, because we know that someone has achieved something great in one area of his life or profession, he must be right about everything. You see this a lot in ads in which Mr. X supposedly accurately predicted the recession, which is meant to have you believe he is a prediction genius, so you better buy his financial advice immediately if not sooner. (Of course, he might never have predicted the recession, or he might have, but it's the only prediction he has got right in fifty years, and so on.)

In the same vein, just because a person has been in the sleep profession for fifty years, is a doctor, or has a great record doesn't make her or him right about everything. Certainly, you would want to pay attention to credentialed professionals, but that doesn't mean they are infallible.

Other biases used by marketers and social media "experts" are:

- o This Hollywood icon swears by the technique
- o The practice has been used for thousands of years
- o Lots of people testify that it worked for them

Recognize that each person is unique and that the most appropriate technique or solution depends on a proper assessment of the situation. It's convenient when we can create energy saving and simple generalities, but they often end up distorting the problem --and the solution.

In short, I am making a plea for a better understanding of sleep challenges by engaging in integrative holistic thinking that recognizes the problems with binary brain and tendencies to assume and overgeneralize. In short, I invite you to explore with a holistic mind and question everything.

Common Misguided Beliefs

Pregnancy:

- o Sleep challenges during pregnancy are expected
- o Sleep loss during pregnancy prepares you for parenting with a new baby
- o Addressing sleep challenges during pregnancy are not necessary and will not make a difference

Infant Sleep:
- o Babies manipulate
- o Babies must sleep the exact hours according to the sleep chart
- o Babies are creating sleep associations and bad habits when rocking, co-sleeping, breast feeding, etc.

- Expect sleep regressions and expect them to be negative
- Co-sleeping with my baby is dangerous
- Babies need to be taught to sleep
- Babies must learn how to self-soothe
- Babies should sleep through the night
- My baby needs to adapt to my schedule
- I need to adapt to my baby's schedule
- Crying is good or bad
- Sleep training is the only alternative in our society when parents are sleep deprived and still need to work

Parenting Sleep:

- Parents are supposed to lose sleep with babies
- Parents do not need to change their lifestyle choices or behaviors
- Babies must adapt to parent's lifestyle
- Parents must adapt to babies
- Sleep deprivation comes with parenting
- My child's sleep issue has nothing to do with me
- My current health and lifestyle choices are not related to my child's sleep

Adult Sleep:

- o I have always been a bad sleeper, so it will always be that way
- o Drinking a glass of wine before bed will help me sleep better
- o I don't need sleep
- o I don't have time to sleep
- o Sleeping with a smartphone or iPad by my bed does not influence sleep
- o What I drink, eat, feel, think and process throughout the day does not affect my night's sleep

So, what I'd like to do is challenge all of this. I'd like to challenge every single one of these beliefs because what I have found is that it's not about being for or against any one belief. Instead, what I have found is that every belief serves a purpose and an intention *during a particular specific circumstance and time.* In one instance co-sleeping may be dangerous, while in another instance it may not. And remember beliefs are not facts. We need to evaluate the evidence for each belief and the purpose it serves, before we can confidently turn it into an effective strategy.

There are so many beliefs that are vague as to be unhelpful. For example, when people feel that babies are manipulative, it's vital to explore what that really means because that is a loaded word. What is the definition of "manipulation"? When we understand a baby's development and what's really happening, we might see "manipulation" in a totally different way.

A lot of times what we perceive, assess and evaluate are not accurate reflections of reality or may just be true for one circumstance but not all. Is it really the case that babies must sleep the exact number of hours according to the sleep chart? When we understand the biology of sleep, the wheel of health and how we are affected by sleep, any rigid rule about child or adult sleep may be limiting. Again, there is so much individual variation that a hard and fast rule can be more misleading than helpful.

This is one of the problems with the evolution of science. When science was only preoccupied with the physical world, it made sense to see facts as certainties. Yes, the sun does come up every day and water boils at 212 degrees Fahrenheit. However, when science moved to considering behavior in addition to the material world, it ran into a problem. Human and animal behavior cannot be described as inevitable facts that can always be predicted, like most of the observable material world. At best, they are probabilities. So, when we conclude that babies "need 16 hours of sleep a day" that is not a "fact" it is a probability that is influenced by many, many variables. However, it has the authority of science and so it seems as if it's a hard and fast rule, but it isn't.

The value of further research is that it helps to define what the factors are that influence the probability that 16 hours is the best amount of sleep. And the issue becomes more complex because effective research can only address a few of the obvious factors at a time and the more factors researched, the more complex the process becomes. It gets to the point where meaningful, definitive research has to be conducted on thousands of subjects over a period of time, which is expensive and often simply not possible.

Another very important issue is that science can typically only give you associations, not causes. So, hypothetically, it might be that babies who only sleep 14 hours a day have more stomach problems. It's natural to think that there's a *causal relationship* between these two variables. Either it's that stomach problems keep the babies awake, or less sleep causes stomach issues, or maybe a bit of both. However, it is also possible, if not likely, that there are other factors causing both problems, like the levels of household stress.

Even research from the very best institutions is limited in its conclusions and implications, because at best, it can show the probability of an association but can't typically answer what the factors are that are responsible for the association. One factor that is likely to be huge in both the design and interpretation of research is the culture.

According to Stephanie Meade in her article "The West's Strange Relationship to Babies and Sleep", in most non-Western societies, babies sleep with their parents, if not in the bed, at least in the same room. So do young children. It is only in industrialized Western countries that sleep has become a compartmentalized, private affair.

In one study (Barry, H., & Paxson, 1971) of 186 nonindustrial societies, 46% of children slept in the same bed as their parents, while 21% slept in a separate bed but in the same room. In other words, in 67% of the cultures around the world, children sleep in the company of others. What is even more significant, in none of those 186 cultures do babies sleep in a separate place before they are at least one year old. The U.S. consistently stands out as a country where babies are routinely placed in their own beds and in their own rooms.

So, views about babies' sleep, from what is the norm to different remedies, are going to vary based on culture, tradition and fear.

In the U.S., there's this approach that focuses on "child independence" – or is it more like adult *independence*? Most couples want to share a bed for sleep. Sure, there may be issues that prevent couples from actually sharing a bed or even a bedroom, but the probability is that most couples want to sleep together.

If we look at adult behavior, there's a very natural tendency for adults to sleep together. They have this arrangement not just because of intimacy, but to feel the closeness of one another while sharing a bed during the entire night. So, is it that strange to have a baby in the same room close to us?

It's not that strange when you really think about it, especially when this child has been developing and growing inside mom's womb for many, many months and is going through the transition of being inside mom to being outside her in the big, wide world.

In the rest of the world, babies don't need their cribs and rooms because everyone expects babies to be close to the mother after birth. They only just came out of the mother's body after all. But most Americans expect them to be in bed all on their own, rather than snuggled up close to the same body where they were inside for nine months. Doesn't that seem odd?

Most of us in the U.S. have been taught by the mainstream to be afraid of bedsharing. However, while there are clear safe bedsharing guidelines provided by Dr. James McKenna, founder of the Mother-Baby Behavioral Sleep Laboratory, many still lack a full understanding of what makes it safe or unsafe. Babies are then separated as a result of this fear, and if they have difficulty with it, we have techniques to manage the "problem". Perhaps the initial premise is wrong?

Part of the problem comes from the western psychological tradition of focusing solely on behavior and fear of safety. The notion of conditioning and habit formation dominated western psychology for most of the twentieth century but has more recently shown to be seriously lacking. The merely behavioral approach doesn't consider the context, let alone the experience of an action. It's not "just a behavior"- it is a lot more meaningful than that. And it is the context and experience that are critical in understanding any behavior, including an infant's sleep. That's what we need to understand.

In other words, the behavioral approaches look at the relation between external cues or stimuli and the behavioral response. However, there is much more going on between the stimulus and the response: perception, context, meaning and so on. Seeing it merely as a relationship between a stimulus and response is too simplistic.

"Between stimulus and response there is a space. In that space is our power to choose our response. In our response lies our growth and our freedom." ~ Viktor Frankl

If we are bonded with someone, do we like to sleep alone? Absent any health or special circumstantial issues that make a bedsharing situation unsafe, typically we want to sleep with those with we love – even our pets! (And many of them love to sleep with us.)

In Japan, where co-sleeping and breastfeeding in the absence of maternal smoking is the cultural norm, rates of sudden infant death syndrome are the lowest in the world. In Italy, you'll see children eating around 9:00 p.m. or running around restaurants at 11 and 12:00 a.m. In Norway, babies are regularly left outside in minus 20-degree weather to sleep and the Yequanna tribe children follow their own inclinations on how to play, how much to eat, when to sleep and so on.

The point is that any one of the generalizations you can make about behavior of any type, including infant sleep, is that it is dangerous to generalize. Remember, behavioral facts aren't "facts", they are probabilities bounded by many unknown factors and influences.

I'm a huge advocate of rhythm, flow and consistency, because I believe they are such important parts of health. Having a schedule and a regular rhythmic flow - one that is in balance, harmony and in tune with nature - is very important. However, that is about flexibility, not rigidity. Being in harmony and balance allows for the most important aspect for all living things: adaptation. Mother Nature is adapting and evolving all the time. It is not the strongest who survive, but the most adaptable. This is an important skill.

"Intelligence is the ability to adapt to change." ~ Stephen Hawking

In our western culture, media, books and authorities have mostly shaped and influenced parent's beliefs about infant sleep – and professional views, too. Parents assume that the information that is being shared by media, books and authorities on infant sleep is the only solution and the real truth and answer. Of course, they are likely to agree with the views that resonate with them the most.

One of the *cognitive biases* that enables us to maintain some level of consistency is *confirmation bias,* in which we will seek out information that supports our views and minimizes or even avoids, conflicting opinions.

This means that "professionals" themselves will cherry pick the "evidence" that confirms their beliefs (which are opinions, not facts). Parents are likely to be drawn to those approaches that they, for one reason or another, agree with. Their decision is usually derived from the cultural narrative that is written from a dominant perspective which excludes many factors that contribute to making an informed decision.

For example, in co-sleeping death articles, you're usually not given specifics about the fact that in most of these cases, the child and the family were not following safe co-sleeping guidelines to begin with or: In any situation, whether you're using the crib, a stroller, a baby product, it's always dangerous to not follow safety guidelines. It is always important that we understand the safety guidelines of anything that we adopt, whether it's a product or something we're implementing in our lifestyle. People who cannot follow safe co-sleeping guidelines should not bedshare.

A lot of families that I have worked with rely on the advice of pediatricians without knowing that pediatrician sleep education is about four to six hours in medical school. Unless the pediatrician has taken extra training and done maybe some self-study, they don't really know that much about child sleep. They are likely to refer to general "standard recommendations of practice", without fully assessing a family's health and lifestyle. So often, the most common advice that parents get from their pediatrician is to separate the child and let the child cry it out.

In NPR's article, "Is Sleeping With Your Baby As Dangerous As Doctors Say?" by Michaeleen Doucleff, doctors in New Zealand have begun taking a more evolved approach to bed sharing called, **The New Zealand strategy**.

> *The results have been tremendous. We've had a 30 percent reduction in mortality since 2010," says Mitchell.*

Specifically, they've been figuring out which babies are at high risk for SIDS. Mitchell has even created a calculator that will give families their personal risk. Then for families at high risk, they're not simply saying, "Don't bed-share" — they've found that many families don't heed that advice — but rather, they're teaching families how to bed-share more safely. For example, they talk about what increases the risk, such as drug use and alcohol use, and they give families a so-called "Moses basket" so that the family can bring the baby into the bed, but the baby is protected from a rollover by this separate sleeping container.

"We're now talking about safer bed-sharing," he says. "And that takes all the steam out of the controversy."

How Perspective & Attitude Greatly Influences Child Sleep

People are not disturbed by things, but by the view they take of them. ~Epictetus

The difference between a mountain and a molehill is your perspective. ~Al Neuharth

When you change your perspective, you change your life.

The following are some examples of child sleep industry terms with limited perspectives influencing how we deal with child sleep challenges.

Sleep Training

According to the Oxford Dictionary "sleep training" is the process of training young children to fall asleep on their own, typically by means of techniques in which the child is left to cry without being comforted, either for gradually increasing periods of time or until they fall asleep.

Sleep training has become a very general term that refers to a variety of approaches including cry it out, no cry and gentle methods to help babies learn to fall asleep by themselves.

People throw out the term "sleep training" very loosely without being specific about what it means and therefore it is left open to one's own interpretation. As a result, it leaves so much room for assumptions and misinterpretations that usually lead to judgement and heated debates.

For this reason, I have not only removed the use of this term from my program and work but when someone uses the term with me, I ask them to please be specific about what they mean so there is no room left for misinterpretations.

Reframing Sleep Training to Sleep Optimizing

Sleep Optimization

I feel a more accurate, positive and beneficial way of describing what many sleep approaches are intending to do is to optimize sleep. Sleep optimization is very powerful.

According to the Merriam-Webster dictionary, "optimization" is an act, process, or methodology of making something (such as a design, system, or decision) as fully perfect, functional, or effective as possible specifically.

Sleep Regression

According to a NY Times Parenting article, "Are Sleep Regressions Real?" by Jessica Wapner, a "sleep regression" refers to a stretch of days or even weeks where babies suddenly don't seem to sleep or nap in the same ways they used to. For many, it feels like a frustrating backpedal on the road to the parenting Valhalla known as Sleeping Through the Night. The concept of infant sleep regressions has been bopping around developmental psychology circles since the 1940s, though the evidence on *when* and *why* they occur is shaky.

Reframing Sleep Regression to Sleep Transition

What seems for most parents and professionals to be a sleep regression setback can instead be perceived as a sleep transition that naturally occurs during child sleep development. Just like the average child begins to take steps around 9 months of age, the child goes through a period of anywhere from 4-6 months during this time of development before he/she fully walks. This similarly happens with sleep development. Just because a child begins to show signs of sleeping optimally doesn't mean they have fully matured and achieved that milestone. So, when a child begins to show signs of sleep maturity, we automatically assume the child's sleep has fully developed and as a result get frustrated when their sleep behavior does not always match the newly formed behavior. However, when we understand our child is naturally developing and transitioning toward a mature stage of sleep, then we will not view their transition as a setback but rather as a natural progression that will include a mix of new and older behaviors.

Sleep Crutch

A "sleep crutch" is the clinical name for a negative sleep association. It's anything that must be done to or for your baby to aid in falling asleep. Some common examples include; nursing, rocking, bottle feeding, walking, bouncing, lying down with your child or rubbing their back to sleep. The idea is that if children use any form of support to fall sleep, a negative sleep association develops and prevents your child from sleeping independently.

Reframing Sleep Crutch to Sleep Anchor

First thing I want you to consider is that needing support for sleep outside of yourself is not necessarily a bad thing, especially if a child is not physically or emotionally or developmentally ready. For example, before a child can walk, he/she needs support along the way in the form of being held or carried by a person or apparatus until their body is ready to begin independently walking on his/her own. The same applies to sleep. So many families have been taught to think that any form of sleep support is negative and will prevent their child from sleeping independently. As a result, they take an all or nothing approach. This results in so much stress, frustration and unrealistic expectations. Rather than perceiving sleep crutches as negative associations, we can empower ourselves, our choices and habits by reframing a sleep crutch to a sleep anchor which is temporarily needed to support a child or an adult toward optimal sleep. Adults who experience sleep challenges may need a sleep anchor to recalibrate their health and lifestyle for optimal sleep.

According to the Vocabulary.com dictionary, the definition of a "crutch" is something you lean on when you're hurt or weak. It can be a physical crutch you use because you broke your leg, or a friend you depend on a bit too much when you're having a tough time. ... A psychological crutch helps you when you need it, or think you do.

So, when we use the word crutch, we already begin with an assumed limitation imposed on our child or an adult. However, if we consider an anchor, an anchor symbolizes security, stability, and being grounded. Understanding that children and adults may need sleep anchors to support their current sleep challenges empowers us to meet our challenges more positively and with less frustration.

The Dreaded Early Riser

The most common limiting perspective amongst parents and professionals in the child sleep industry is that of early risers.

So many parents and professionals view early rising as a problem even if a child is meeting their total number of daily sleep requirements.

But is early rising so bad? While there could be so many reasons of early rising (due to an imbalance which should be addressed), the truth is that some children are biologically wired to rise early. It is not only important to take this into consideration, but recognize that as we age, science positively backs up early rising, citing so many benefits found through extensive research.

Many parents dread early rising - not because it has affected their child's sleep or health - but because they themselves are not early risers or because they have beliefs that early rising is a problem. Rather than forcing a child who is wired to rise early to adapt to your schedule, perhaps we can consider the benefits early rising may have for our own sleep habits and as a result make changes to our own lifestyle that will be more beneficial to us and suitable for the natural rhythm wired in our children. Now, you may be thinking what happens if the mother is a night owl and her child an early bird? Whose biological wiring gets priority? Are adults expected to re-wire themselves to accommodate their baby? The answer is you both can get priority when you follow a team approach. I elaborate more on the team led approach in my Parental Authority vs. Parental Leadership chapter further into the book. There is not one solution that will fit each case. In every challenge lies an opportunity. When we can let go of our limiting beliefs, expectations, take space and embrace a team perspective, the solution we need to meet both our needs and our child's needs will become clear.

Sleep Education & Support During Pregnancy

I'm a huge advocate for starting sleep education and support during pregnancy.

A healthy mom equals a healthy baby. Sleep supports all the vital components of healthy human function. Pregnancy is a perfect time to prepare and establish new rest and sleep habits for healthy sleep to continue long after the baby arrives, and for the rest of her and her baby's life.

As I shared during my introduction, when I first came into the field of child sleep, I was surprised that most of the coaching for infant and child sleep didn't happen until at least the fourth month or even later. For me, there are some very compelling reasons for working with pregnant moms and families. Before the baby arrives, and for that very reason, I have ensured that the sleep professionals I train begin supporting families during pregnancy.

First, as mentioned earlier in my book, there's a high percentage (78%) of pregnant women experiencing sleep challenges of some kind.

Sleep disturbances are common during pregnancy and can be risk factors for several serious pregnancy-related sleep disorders. These can be debilitating and influence the experience of pregnancy and the preparation for welcoming a new family member. On their own, pregnancy sleep issues are enough of a reason to address sleep and rest at this stage. This is critical, because the physiological and emotional state of the mother is experienced by the baby in the womb. Poor sleep and little rest will not only lead to physiological issues with the mother-to-be, but potentially her baby, too. Lack of sleep and rest also lead to an increase in stress, which can impact the health of mother and baby. And it's quite possible that the baby is learning about sleep and cycles, which if disrupted, might influence the baby's natural sleep patterns, too. It is likely that the fetus is influenced by these rhythms of nature. According to article, "Prenatal stress changes brain connectivity in-utero", from the Cognitive Neuroscience Society, a mother's stress during pregnancy changes neural connectivity in the brain of her unborn child. Researchers found that mothers reporting high stress had fetuses with a reduced efficiency in how their neural functional systems are organized. It is the first time, imaging has shown a direct influence of maternal stress on fetal brain development, independent of influences of the postnatal environment.

Second, in addition to not prioritizing rest during the day, many expecting families don't understand the importance of sleep and how their sleep habits are influencing their unborn child. Waiting until the baby has already arrived is a bit like learning to use the fire extinguisher when a fire breaks out. It's far better to reflect about the issues surrounding sleep and rest, before you are faced with that problem. For one thing, you're likely to be less tired and more focused.

Third, addressing sleep issues before a baby arrives allows all family members to be involved and address their own needs. It's like assembling the team and going to Spring Training, something you want to do before the season starts.

Fourth, when you inform and educate a family before the baby arrives, the focus is not on the baby's disrupted sleep, but family sleep and rest patterns. This is very beneficial as you are then less likely to get hung up on baby sleep theories and methods and have a more holistic approach to family sleep, rather than a misguided focus on just the baby's sleep.

Fifth is prevention of postpartum depression and anxiety.

It wasn't until about a century ago that the family unit consisted of two parents or a single parent. The norm was that aunts, uncles, grandparents, cousins and friends helped to raise a child. The number of responsibilities and stress placed on today's parent makes them more vulnerable and susceptible to postpartum depression and anxiety.

According to Dr. Harvey Karp, "Three sources of stress that are common triggers for PPD and are amenable to a specific highly effective intervention: exhaustion, persistent infant crying, and unsupportive partners

The good news is that with education and preparation, one greatly minimizes the risk of experiencing PPD.

Now, let's look a bit closer at why pregnant women experience sleep challenges. There are various reasons for disrupted sleep during pregnancy.

Hormonal changes affect sleep. Sleep is dependent on the daily fluctuation of certain hormones. For example, progesterone induces sleepiness and increased levels can mean daytime sleepiness and sleep for pregnant women, which can disrupt nighttime sleeping. Hormonal changes can also lead to more nighttime urination and muscle fatigue which, can disrupt sleep. Muscle fatigue can also increase the risk of obstructive sleep apnea, which can have a very detrimental effect on sleep quality and leave you feeling very drowsy the following day.

Pregnancy is an emotional and potentially stressful time, as parents prepare for a major life-changing event. Most pregnant women do not rest during the day. Their excitement and their stress can equally be disruptive to sleep. This is especially true of first-time parents, as the impending changes to their lives and relationships can create anxiety.

Nausea and physical discomfort also disrupt sleep, along with other pregnancy-enhanced conditions like restless legs syndrome (RLS). Mauro Manconi, MD, of the Sleep Disorders Center at Vita-Salute University in Milan, Italy, and colleagues, studied pregnancy and restless leg syndrome using a recently revised international definition of the condition. In one study of more than 600 pregnant women, more than 25% of them experienced RLS. Another problem is heartburn, or gastroesophageal reflux (GERD). According to the book, *Practical Gastroenterology and Hepatology Board Review Toolkit* GERD is common in pregnancy. Heartburn is experienced by 30- 50% of pregnant women, though the incidence may be as high as 80%.

As mentioned above, sleep apnea is more common during pregnancy and needs to be taken seriously. It is associated not just with difficulties for the pregnant woman, but other complications such as gestational hypertension, preeclampsia and low birth weight. Research at the University of California at San Francisco found that women who *slept less than 6 hours per night had longer labors and were almost five times more likely to have cesarean deliveries.*

Common sleep problems in pregnancy may include:

Insomnia – symptoms include difficulty falling asleep, staying asleep, or waking up too early or feeling unrefreshed. It can also be caused by physical manifestations of pregnancy such as nausea, back pain and fetal movements.

Restless legs syndrome (RLS) - symptoms of RLS include unpleasant feelings in the legs, like tingling and aching. Worse at night, these discomforts can be relieved by stretching or movement.

Sleep apnea – sleep apnea is a sleep disorder in which breathing is repeatedly interrupted during sleep. A noticeable feature of sleep apnea is heavy snoring accompanied by long pauses, and then gasping or choking during sleep.

Nocturnal gastroesophageal reflux (nighttime GERD) – GERD, also known as heartburn, is considered a normal part of pregnancy. However, nighttime symptoms of GERD can damage the esophagus and disrupt sleep during pregnancy.

Frequent nighttime urination – the frequent need to urinate at night is a common feature of pregnancy and can result in loss of sleep.

Good quality sleep and feeling well-rested during pregnancy is a massive blessing. When mom is rested and feels better about herself, her body and mind function more optimally. As a result, she provides many benefits to her baby's function and natural rhythms. It is also likely to strengthen the bond between her and her baby during her pregnancy, as she will be less stressed and more connected to her baby, while preparing emotionally and physically for a more optimal delivery.

By supporting a pregnant woman (and her partner or whoever is involved) to face sleep challenges, the family has an opportunity to evaluate their quality of life and the choices they are making. The chances are that the family is set up for more effective collaboration and understanding on this issue, which will unquestionably prepare and help once the baby has arrived. There are several ways that pregnant women and their families can prepare during this stage. Much of it will be through education, strengthening consciousness, instilling a holistic mindset, and supporting them with health and lifestyle changes where sleep becomes a value and priority for the whole family.

It's also a great opportunity to assess expectations, beliefs, commitment levels, the state of their consciousness, overall well-being, self-confidence, intuitive abilities, knowledge and support systems.

Not only will family members be more receptive to these changes before the birth, but they won't have to learn during crisis mode - when their baby is having difficulty sleeping - keeping the household awake, too.

As wisely advised by Sadhguru, learning to read our "user's manual" is key to understanding and optimally resolving any challenge we face. He says, *"It is your inability to manage your own system that causes this problem. Assume control over your own being, and everything will be fine. The user's manual is written within you."*

Below are some general tips for pregnancy-related sleep that can further support learning and understanding around sleep challenges. Please know that a full evaluation is needed in order to properly support your (or your clients) specific needs with customized solutions.

Also keep in mind that ultimately, your body carries within it all this intelligence. Through slowing down your mind, you will gain clarity and be guided toward the next steps and solutions that are best for you.

Evaluate Your Lifestyle, Health History and Family History

There are so many forces that affect sleep. In order to get to the root of the challenge, we must first investigate the strongest forces that affect sleep in order to first rule those "causes" out. Rarely is there just one main "problem" or factor. Often there are many forces acting upon a family that prevent them from getting good sleep. Evaluating your lifestyle, health and family history provide important details and clues that lead to discovering the root of your sleep challenge.

Plan, schedule and prioritize sleep

You deserve it! Most people prioritize and schedule everything else but their sleep. Prioritizing, planning and scheduling your sleep will support your health and ability to be more productive in all areas of your life.

Exercise regularly

Upon approval from your healthcare provider, exercise regularly for at least 30 minutes per day and choose the appropriate exercise suitable for your needs, level, stage of pregnancy and current state of health.

Process feelings

It is not uncommon to have trouble sleeping due to overwhelming emotions like fear, anxiety, anger, sadness, grief, depression, excitement taking over. Give yourself permission to ask and receive support to process out these feelings, understand the root of them and not avoid or resist them.

Trust and develop a strong connection with your body

Our body gives us signals indicating it needs rest or sleep that we often ignore for many reasons - from managing responsibilities to entertainment. As we develop a keen sense of awareness of our body and its needs, we will have the ability to know when and how much sleep and rest we need. Trust that when we prioritize and care for our body's need to rest and sleep, everything else will be taken care of too.

Keep your room very dark

If you need to get up to use the bathroom at night, rather than turning on bright lights, use a small nightlight instead of turning on the light to use the bathroom — this will be less arousing and help you return to sleep more quickly. Using just enough light for you to see, and not be too overstimulating to the eye and sleep cycle, will help you maintain a relaxed state.

According to the Live Science article, "How Blue LEDs Affect Sleep" by Alina Bradford, when artificial light is added to a human's day, the body's natural rhythms become confused. The retina can now receive light no matter what time of day it is, so the body doesn't know when to get ready for sleep. A study published in the Endocrine Society's Journal of Clinical

Endocrinology & Metabolism found that, when compared with dim light, exposure to room light during the night suppressed melatonin by around 85 percent in trials.

Keep a journal and pen handy by your bedside

If you have trouble falling asleep because your mind is racing, or if you wake up with too many thoughts and are unable to go back to sleep, consider doing some journaling before crawling into bed at night or when woken up at night to clear the mind so there is no residue.

Be aware of your breathing pattern and engage in breathing exercises

Focus on deepening your breath, calming your nervous system and slowing down your mind. Our body needs to be in a parasympathetic state (or "rest and digest") for sleep. Our breath is the link between our body and our mind.

Invite downtime and enjoy spending time with yourself

Welcome downtime and get accustomed to feeling rested. Our bodies are designed to be at ease and rest and not in a constant state of tension. Engage in activities regularly that are relaxing and letting go of stress. Some examples: include nature walks, hiking, yoga, meditation, journaling, massage, etc. You can use smartphone apps (like the CALM app) to assist you or you can try Yoga Nidra (aka "sleep yoga")." According to Swami Satyananda, one hour of Yoga Nidra is as restful as a few hours of quality sleep.

Invite regularity

Regularity is one of the keys to good sleep. Your mind and body thrive on regularity. When you stick to a similar sleep schedule every night, your body can find its natural rhythm and settle into a regular sleep-wake cycle. It does not have to be rigid, but consistent.

Dim lights or turn on "night shift" mode

Dim all lights and turn your display and brightness setting to "night shift" mode for your computer and smart phone screens at least an hour or two before bed. Install dimmer switches on lights where possible. Candlelight is best for illuminating the house during the hours before bedtime, and many find it to be very relaxing.

Establish firm boundaries for bedtime

Make your bedroom a sanctuary for relaxation and sleep. Try not to do work, watch television, or any other activity outside of sleep and sex.

Remove EMFs

Remove any equipment that has electromagnetic fields (or EMFs). Studies have shown prolonged exposure can suppress the immune system and disrupt sleep. According to the article in Advances in Biology, "Health Implications of Electromagnetic Fields, Mechanisms of Action, and Research Needs", by Sarika Singh and Neeru Kapoor, several human and animal studies conducted thus far have suggested decrease in melatonin after EMF exposure.

Evaluate bedroom air quality

Your bedroom air quality may be affecting your sleep. Make sure your room is well-ventilated and clear of air pollutants such as dust, air fresheners, pet dander, perfumes, etc.

Get natural unfiltered sunlight

Getting at least fifteen minutes of unfiltered sunlight in your eyes first thing in the morning will send a strong message to your pineal gland and your internal clock. In the warmer months or in warmer climates, getting sunlight on a good portion of your skin in the morning as well will help with sleep. Morning sunlight strengthens your natural circadian rhythms. It works wonders. According to the article, "The importance of morning sunlight for better sleep" by Amelia Willson,

> By exposing your eyes to this bright light early in the morning, you signal to your brain that it's time to suppress melatonin production. In response, your brain will increase cortisol production. Cortisol and melatonin operate indirectly to each other. Cortisol is popularly known your stress hormone. While too-high levels of cortisol can be dangerous, in healthy amounts cortisol is good for you. This activating hormone energizes your body and prepares you to meet the day.
>
> Besides light, the sun also emits a lot of warmth. Morning sunlight can warm your body up, facilitating your natural thermoregulation process and aiding cortisol production.
>
> Finally, sunlight affects yet another hormone related to sleep. Greater exposure to sunlight is associated with a

release in serotonin. Serotonin plays an important role in melatonin production, as your pineal gland metabolizes serotonin into melatonin.

Serotonin is also known as the "happy" hormone for its ability to lift mood. In fact, sunlight has such an effect on your mood, that specialized light therapy lamps are used to treat people with seasonal depression and related sleep disorders. These lamps are designed to mimic natural sunlight, without the harmful UV rays.

Just be mindful to prevent overexposure if you plan on staying in the sun for a long time. You can try going without sunscreen for just the first 10–30 minutes, depending on how sensitive your skin is to sunlight, and apply sunscreen before you start burning.

Adjust temperature and evaluate air quality

Keep the temperature between 68 and 72 degrees. Our bodies naturally drop in temperature at night and so keeping the bedroom environment a few degrees cooler, helps us deepen our sleep. According to Dr. Christopher Winter, Medical Director at Charlottesville Neurology & Sleep Medicine, the REM cycle is sensitive to extreme temperatures; sleeping in temperatures above 75 degrees or below 54 degrees can have a negative impact on the brain's ability to complete the REM cycle. When it comes to air quality, a 2015 study conducted at the Technical University of Denmark asked participants to sleep for one week each in differently ventilated bedrooms, to assess the effects of fresh air on sleep. The researchers found that when air was able to move about the room and ventilate, the subjects' sleep quality improved. Participants reported feeling better the next day and scored objectively higher on a test of logical thinking after sleeping in the well-ventilated room.

Use sleeping aids

Use sleeping aids like sleep pillows or a mattress topper for your comfort and support. Have a mattress, mattress topper, or sleeping pillow that is equipped to support your posture. Experiment with them to find the best ones suitable for you.

Adjust sleep position

Pillows and positioning can aid or hinder strong circulation and blood supply needed for fetal development. Most medical birth professionals say that lying on your left side is best because although while lying on your right side may not harm the baby during pregnancy, your uterus puts pressure on the liver. Lying on your back during pregnancy puts pressure on the inferior vena cava, cutting off blood supply. While lying on your front during pregnancy may be a rare occurrence after the first trimester, it places pressure on the womb, putting the baby at risk. When sleeping, lie on your left side with your knees and hips bent. Place pillows between your knees, under your abdomen and behind your back. This may take pressure off your lower back.

Hydrate

Drink lots of fluids during the day, especially a quality, electrolyte-rich mineral water. But cut down on the amount you drink in the hours before bedtime. According to the National Sleep Foundation,

> *Hydration plays a critical role in how well (or not) you sleep at night. Understanding the impact of your daily fluid intake on your nighttime slumber will go a long way to improving the quality of your sleep.*

> *Dehydration causes your mouth and nasal passages to become dry, setting you up for sleep-disruptive snoring and a parched throat and hoarseness in the morning.*

A lack of pre-bed fluids can also lead to nocturnal leg cramps that may keep you awake. In addition to the frustration of fragmented sleep, being dehydrated during night can compromise your alertness, energy, and cognitive performance the following day.

Eat light meals and easily digested foods before bed

Eat only light meals before bed and familiarize yourself with anti-sleep and pro-sleep foods, that I cover in the chapter on The Power and Influence of Nutrition for Sleep, in order to avoid sleep disruption and encourage deep sleep.

Eat foods that are more easily digestible, like blended foods and fruits with unprocessed fats, and keep your portion sizes small as you approach bedtime.

Eliminate all stimulants from your diet

This includes caffeine, chocolate, and spices of all kinds. It is also critical to eliminate foods that are stimulating and irritating to the digestive system just by their very nature—foods like grains, beans, and dairy. This is even more essential late in the day. Grains tend to bind with the cholesterol in your gut that is needed to produce sleep-inducing hormones and other necessary cofactors. MSG a.k.a. monosodium glutamate, is a neurotoxin you should avoid. It is hidden in all sorts of products nowadays under many different names like "textured vegetable protein", "hydrolyzed vegetable protein", and "yeast extract" to name a few. One should also be careful of taking vitamin supplements in the evening as they can have a stimulating effect, and in many cases, they are like a chemistry experiment. It's probably best to take them in the morning or early afternoon if possible.

Know the difference between folic acid and folate

It is common for doctors to advise pregnant women to take lots of folic acid. Too little or too much folic acid can disrupt sleep as well as cause other health related issues. According to the American Pregnancy Association, people often use folic acid and folate interchangeably as they are both forms of vitamin B9 but in fact there is an important difference. Folic acid is the synthesized version that is commonly used in processed foods and supplements such as wheat products, like breads and pastas. Folate can be found in whole foods such as leafy vegetables, eggs, and citrus fruits. It is estimated that between 25 and 60 percent of the population have a variation in one of their MTHFR genes that negatively impacts their ability to convert folic acid (the synthetic version of B9). As such women taking folic acid may not be absorbing their B vitamins as expected.

And when the body can't break it down and use it, it becomes depleted in this critical B vitamin, and the body treats the synthetic form as a toxin. This results for some in symptoms like weight gain and eventual obesity, or the toxin can also be funneled away into the joints where it manifests as arthritis.

The American Pregnancy Association says for this reason, it's preferable to take folate either from whole food sources or supplements that containing the natural form of active folate instead of synthesized folic acid whenever possible.

Healthy blood sugar levels

Blood sugar has a huge impact on sleep quality. Observe your body's reaction to high sugar foods and the impacts they have on mood and fatigue. Strive to keep your blood sugar level stable to increase energy, ward off fatigue, and sleep better at night.

Establish healthy gut flora

Something else to consider is your gut. It is important to establish healthy gut flora and then leave it alone. Many researchers are now strongly linking the cyclical die-off of bacteria in the gut with sleep cycles.

According to the article in the US National Library of Medicine, National Library of Health, "The Role of Microbiome in Insomnia, Circadian Disturbance and Depression", numerous studies have suggested that the incidence of insomnia and depressive disorder are linked to biological rhythms, immune function, and nutrient metabolism, but the exact mechanism is not yet clear. There is considerable evidence showing that the gut microbiome not only affects the digestive, metabolic, and immune functions of the host but also regulates host sleep and mental states through the microbiome-gut-brain axis.

Reduce stress

Listening to your body and giving it what it needs will naturally reduce stress. Some examples may include sleeping longer, taking naps, or committing to engaging in relaxing daily activities. Sleep helps to balance stress hormones. When feeling anxious and/or stressed, your nervous system causes physiological changes in your body. The brain's perception of stress signals the release of stress hormones, like adrenaline and cortisol, into the bloodstream. This causes your body to react in a "fight-or-flight" response. When this state is activated, your digestive system slows down, preventing essential nutrients from being absorbed. Your muscles also become very tense, making you more susceptible to injuries, as well as making it more difficult to think clearly.

"Green" your sleeping environment

"Greening" your sleep environment is essential to diminish the risks of toxic exposures which can compromise your immune system leading to a host of possible health issues. A few tips for "Greening" a sleep environment include: removing disruptive items (such as products with fragrances and items that may emit EMFs), leaving shoes at the door, using non-toxic cleaners, using indoor plants that clean the air, improving ventilation, removing pet dander or pets from your bedroom environment and washing bed-sheets, linens, pillowcases, and pajamas with non-toxic laundry detergent.

Be mindful of environment noise

Nighttime noises from your internal and external environment can disrupt sleep such ass traffic, dogs barking, partner snoring, toilet running, faucet dripping, bed frame creaking, etc. Be mindful of them and if they are out of your control, invest in a quality white noise machine or customized ear plugs.

Additional considerations about sleep

- Pets can be noisy and disrupt sleep. For example, cats or dogs may be active at night. Remove any toys or jingly collars.

- Snoring is very common during pregnancy, but if you have pauses in your breathing associated with your snoring, you should be screened for sleep apnea. Also, have your blood pressure and urine protein checked— especially if you have swollen ankles or headaches.

- If you develop RLS, you should be evaluated for iron or folate deficiency.

- Add daytime naps as necessary, but reduce them or nap earlier in the day if you have difficulty falling asleep at night.

- Check your magnesium levels. According to Healthline's article, "7 Signs and Symptoms of Magnesium Deficiency", while less than 2% of Americans have been estimated to experience magnesium deficiency, one study suggests that up to 75% are not meeting their recommended intake. Magnesium, also known as "nature's tranquilizer", can be a basic treatment for insomnia and helps with relaxation and sleep.

Managing stress during pregnancy

With our modern-day culture and expectations, the average person is juggling quite a bit and as a result, experiencing an overwhelming amount of stimulation and stress. Incorporating relaxation and rest into your daily life is the perfect complement to healthy sleep and your overall health.

Babies exposed to a variety of stress hormones, toxins and malnutrition inside the womb may develop a host of problems during their fetal growth and after they are born. Their bodies have to undergo certain biological changes in order to cope with a high-stress environment. These physiological changes can lead to premature labor or even complications during labor.

In October of 2009, The UK Times reported new research that shows exactly how stress can harm a baby's development, and how that stress can lead to long-term problems.

According to research by Vivette Glover, a professor of perinatal psychobiology, maternal anxiety affects the placenta by reducing the activity of the main barrier enzyme that hinders the hormone cortisol from reaching the fetus. The babies of women who were stressed during pregnancy had lower birth weights, lower IQs, slower cognitive development, and more anxiety than those born to the other women in the study.

Managing sleep and stress is key during and after pregnancy and the two have a reciprocal relationship. Stress interrupts sleep as cortisol levels that normally drop in the evening hours, stay high. Quality sleep helps to defuse the stress-induced changes. As a result, reducing stress and integrating relaxation into your daily lifestyle are the perfect complement to healthy sleep, overall health, and the health of your baby.

How can women cope, and prevent stress and anxiety?

When I was pregnant, I found a few things essential to my (and my baby's) well-being.

Acceptance

I had to accept and feel comfortable with my feelings, and not try to resist them. It is perfectly normal to have some doubts or fears surrounding labor, especially if you are a first-time parent. Once you allow and invite your feelings to be present, you will be able to take the steps you need to process them, take care of yourself and your baby, while reducing — if not eliminating — stress altogether.

Support

I sought support. This could be through an expectant mom's group, a childbirth education class, or a qualified professional — such as a birth doula. By working with a birth doula, attending a birth education class or expectant moms group, you can prevent or reduce stress levels dramatically. Birth doulas are trained to provide expectant moms emotional and physical support in preparation for labor and are also present during labor for support. Childbirth education classes are designed to inform expectant mothers of their options for labor and birth and prepare them for the journey. An expectant moms group can also be another great resource; you will be able to relate to and share all the uncertainties and fears you have with other women who are going through the same process.

Sleep and relaxation

I made it a priority to rest daily. It is so important to make sure you are getting as much sleep as your body needs, as well as taking some downtime throughout the day. Your body repairs itself during sleep and works to restore any imbalances that are occurring. When you compromise sleep, you become more susceptible to stress, as your immune system must work harder to maintain proper levels of functioning throughout the day. Also consider taking some downtime through a yoga or meditation class, a brisk walk, bubble bath, or even by lightening your workload.

Nutrition

Nutrition plays a very powerful role in both coping with and the prevention of stress while I was pregnant. Caffeine, sugar and processed foods can trigger stress, so it is best to avoid them. Eat whole, fresh organic foods: fruits, vegetables, protein, and healthy fats that are easy to digest, and contain bio-available nutrients that are especially high in B vitamins and minerals. Exposure to sunshine for a few minutes of day will help your body absorb these nutrients. Of course, be sure to consult your midwife, doctor or nutritionist for your specific dietary needs.

Develop a keen sense of awareness

When we develop a keen sense of awareness, we will naturally do whatever we need to do to support our wellbeing. When we are fully conscious, we are clear and powerful to handle any challenge. Consciousness is the light that dispels the darkness.

The greatest gift we can begin giving ourselves and our babies during pregnancy is developing a keen sense of awareness. This means spending time going within. For many of us this may seem challenging at first but when you understand the enormous benefits and potential, you will be driven to do it. Take baby steps. Start with a few minutes each day and increase time as your body and mind become accustomed and begin to feel a sense of well-being from it.

Have fun and celebrate

It's hard to be stressed when you are having fun. During pregnancy with so much going on, it is easy to forget to have fun and celebrate the journey. For example, treat yourself to a spa day or a photoshoot. Hang out with other expecting moms over lunch, dinner or a movie. Participate in prenatal exercise classes like prenatal dance or yoga.

Should you seek medical help or therapy?

If you have tried everything and find yourself with unknown causes of symptoms, or feeling helpless or depressed, it's always best to seek medical attention or therapy. There are many professionals who are dedicated and committed to supporting you through your journey and can provide you and your little one on board with the necessary help.

Now that we have covered an overview of pregnancy sleep, we will move on to child sleep. Let's begin with the history of child sleep and sleep training.

History of Child Sleep & Sleep Training

The history of child sleep and child sleep training is very interesting. In the Industrial Revolution in the 18th century, mothers were warned not to spoil their children. If you think about it, the Industrial Revolution is not too long ago. Nonetheless, co-sleeping was a very common practice up until the 19th century even in the industrialized west.

Cribs were moved to another room if the home was large enough. With infants sleeping alone, it was easy for parents to follow the *cry it out* advice even if it went against their gut instinct. The cultural message created a fear of raising demanding monsters. In the 20th century, there was a detached method introduced where bottle feeding replaced breastfeeding during the sleep *cry it out* phase.

Dr. Luther Emmet Holt, an American pediatrician and child-rearing expert, was the first person to make the cry it out approach explicit in 1894. Then behavioral psychologist, John B. Watson, a leader in behaviorism, followed up in 1928 with advice that basically supported Dr. Luther Emmet Holt and created schedules as parent-led regimens. Dr. Benjamin Spock came out in the 1940s and '50s with his huge book on child rearing and parenting. Dr Richard Ferber followed with his book, "Solve Your Child's Sleep Problems" in 1985, Dr Marc Weissbluth followed with his book, "Health Sleep Habits, Happy Child" in 1987, Elizabeth Pantley followed with her book, "The No Cry Sleep Solution in 2002, and so on. This list is almost endless. Then in 2012, I introduced the first holistic professional training program for adult and child sleep consultants via my company, the International Parenting & Health Institute. Today we are represented in 46 countries and in 10 languages with high success rates from professionals and their clients implementing my approach.

Since then and more recently, there are others who are coming forward and sharing their versions of a holistic approach as well. It's wonderful to see how we are now entering into this stage, this next evolution of adult and child sleep, with a deeper and clearer understanding of sleep challenges. There's really not just one right way for everyone. It depends on a number of factors.

These trends reflect what is happening in behavioral science in general. There's a recognition that the behavioral approach is too limited in its scope and philosophy. It came from a cultural philosophy of independence that overlooked critical factors and the huge role of interdependency, that is much more valued in many other sociocentric (as opposed to egocentric) cultures.

These limitations have misled the public. Yes, it would be easier if there was a standard set of rules that applied to every child and every adult in every circumstance, but it simply doesn't work that way.

I have worked with families where their child is healthy; they're developing well. When you look at the full number of hours that they're sleeping in a 24-hour period, it's right in the "range". There's really nothing that stands out as a red flag. Yet, the parents have interpreted the child's sleep behavior as somehow "out of the norm". And, of course, I have worked with families who were very concerned - unreasonably so - because their child did not fit into the box of latest standards, schedules or requirements as listed in their book. It's incredible to me how parents insist that there's a problem, where none seems evident.

In the same vein, I have worked with families whose child is waking up multiple times in the night. Prior to working with me, they had resorted to sleep training to get their child to sleep. However, when sleep training did not work, they searched deeper for answers. Further investigation revealed that their child was waking up due to a food tolerance, nutritional deficiency, unresolved birth trauma or many other reasons. I have even worked with families whose child had sleep challenges simply because the parents were hyper-focused on getting their child to sleep.

It's not just parents who are rigid. Most mainstream sleep consultants I have come across are very fixed in their thinking. They swear by inflexible structures and scientific standards. Instead of evaluating someone's entire health and lifestyle, they make assumptions, resulting in a one-size-fits-all method being prescribed. This undoubtedly carries with it many limitations. For example, to expect every child under the age of one should sleep independently and through the night is completely unrealistic. Or to say that every child at six months of age should sleep the same number of hours each night and at the same exact times is also unrealistic.

You'd have to say that every child's circumstances, history, health, family, environment, circadian rhythm, etc. must also be the same.

This brings me to Dr. Gwen Dewar, founder of www.parentingscience.com

She says:

> *Everybody knows that babies need more sleep than older children do. But how much? When I began researching baby sleep requirements, I assumed that those authoritative charts we see published everywhere—the ones telling us that the average newborn needs 16 hours of sleep, for example—were based on scientifically-established, biological needs. I figured that somebody must have identified a link between, say, a certain minimum number of sleep hours and optimal rates of childhood growth. Or between sleep hours and rates of infection. I was wrong. It turns out that scientists know relatively little about baby sleep requirements. The sleep charts that you see in parenting books and websites are based on*

how much time parents—typically, Western parents—say their babies spend sleeping. For instance, studies of Australian babies reveal that the average newborn gets about 16-17 hours of sleep over a 24-hour period. Babies aged 4-6 months average 14 hours.

There has been a lot of recent research, digging deeper into the issue of average sleep times for infants. These estimates have fluctuated and expanded somewhat over the years, but again, the requirements really depend on so many factors that one should not rely on statistics alone.

Therefore, I present you with a revolutionary way to meet your sleep challenges, fueled by a multicultural yet bio-individualized approach, that empowers you to connect with your inner guidance system, support your own well-being and strengthen your family connection.

Do Children Need to Be Trained to Sleep?

A popular misconception that you may hear is that children need to be trained to sleep, do not know how to sleep and that they need to learn and be taught how to sleep.

Sleep is a natural and necessary function, much like elimination is a natural function and feeding is a natural function. Just like walking has natural stages of child development, so does sleep. In the same way not every child will walk exactly at the same age or begin eating solids at the same age, we cannot expect every child to sleep through the night and be independent at the same age.

While there is an average age estimate of when developmental milestones are reached, it is just an average estimate and as we also know some children are developmentally delayed and some are developmentally advanced.

Our body, as dictated by nature, is designed to sleep. Children experience developmental milestones with sleep in the same way they develop skills to walk, talk, etc. So, it is not that a child needs to learn to sleep as much as it is a child needs the proper set up, support and environment so sleep development can take its natural course. As a result, what we need to understand is what is getting in the way of this natural function.

There are several things that get in the way of child sleep: medical, environmental, nutritional, physical, emotional and many other external and internal factors. One area that is often not considered is how much we as parents, and as professionals, can get in the way of children's sleep.

One only must consider our current culture and society.

Consider your energy, drive, mood, priorities and lifestyle before and after having your child. Are you constantly on the go? Do you ever give yourself a chance to pause, slow down or even stop? If you're not focused on your extensive to do list, do you consider yourself a failure? Do you feel that you always must be productive to be fulfilled? Do you feel guilty if you take some time out for yourself? Is there any semblance of balance in your life? At the end of the day are you rested and ready for restorative sleep or are you exhausted and about to collapse? What example are you setting and what energy are you creating in your home environment?

Whether we like it or not, our children will model and respond to what we do.

"If you're going to hold yourself up to your children, hold yourself up as a warning not an example." ~ George Bernard Shaw

Being part of a stressful household is stressful.

Interdependence, not independence, is the name of the game. Our children are naturally integrating and co-existing with us. We're all co-existing and we're all naturally adapting to each other's energies.

There is a lot of research that says during the first seven years of a child's life, the child is effectively in a hypnotic state. They're basically downloading all these programs, just absorbing and taking in. They are training their brains to adapt to the situations in which they find themselves. They're designed to do that intelligently so that they can also learn how to survive and function. So, we're huge role models for them, and how we are living our lives and what we are modeling for our children are going to be direct and massive influences in their lives.

And if we're going, going, going, turned on all the time, and we're not allowing ourselves to slow down and pause, or if we're not teaching ourselves and learning how to integrate relaxation and rest into our own lifestyle, how can we expect our children to do the same?

We've been conditioned to "go, go, go". We've been conditioned to believe that our children can't sleep and don't want to sleep. We've been taught that we must rely on authorities, experts and one-size-fits-all methods to tell us how to sleep. In reality, the best that experts and professionals can do is shine a light on the areas of our lives that are limiting us and our children's ability to sleep. This includes empowering ourselves to develop a stronger connection with our bodies, slowing down, supporting, inspiring, and encouraging ourselves to make healthy changes so that we can feel motivated to take action, while having the confidence to know that we can sleep and that our children can sleep.

We can relate this to modern-day conveniences. How often are we introduced to technologies that will allow our current modern lifestyles to be even more convenient? They theoretically allow us to get more work done and allow us to make more money.

Quite often modern-day technologies have been used, not necessarily to complement our lifestyles, but to replace our parenting. While modern-day technology can be used beneficially to complement our lifestyles, we absolutely need to pay attention when technology begins to replace human connection and development.

There is neither a crib, doll, nor gadget that is going to replace the natural heart-to-heart, parent to child connection. As close as we probably get to that, it's never going to be the same thing. So again, it's not about avoiding technology; it's about working with it in a way that complements and benefits our lifestyle.

Now, something to consider for a moment is whether a child really needs sleep training, or we do? For example, how often do we want our child to sleep because we have a need to fulfill?

We often say I need to make that phone call! I need to get that work project done! I need to relax. I need to get this done and that done while my child sleeps. So, the child getting to sleep becomes more about us and our needs, rather than the child's needs.

Now, I'm not suggesting ignoring your needs. It's not about ignoring your needs. It's about understanding that when we're co-existing in a family unit, everybody's needs are important. Acknowledging when our need is overriding our child's need helps us understand how we might be getting in the way of our children's ability to sleep. Isn't it funny how that happens? It's when we need to get our child to sleep the most that they don't sleep!

As a result, it's helpful to take a step back and ask ourselves: "Why am I needing my child to sleep, and do I have to revisit that and have another way of approaching the situation?"

What I have found is that sleep training, or re-training, really needs to start with parents and professionals. We can provide further help once we understand that we don't need to teach or train our children how to sleep, and that it's about learning what's getting in the way of sleep, which sometimes, turns out to be us.

Yes, the "problem" could be medical environmental, physical, emotional, or any number of factors. But we don't often see our behaviors and lifestyles as big factors in holding back our child from sleeping. Once we start to wake up to that, not only do we have a tremendous opportunity to get our child to sleep, but we also get the rest that we, as well as the whole family, need. We have an opportunity to evolve to another level of personal growth, of understanding. When we're well-rested, we feel better, we're more conscious, connected, more effective problem solvers and we can enjoy life more.

This is one of the many reasons why I love the world of sleep, because sleep is not just about recharging and restoring our bodies. Sleep can also be a window to discovering something much deeper and greater that exists within all of us and that is ready to be a part of a huge evolution in our humanity.

In Yolanda Smith's article "Function of Sleep" on News Medical Life Science, she writes:

It is believed that sleeping and dreaming help in the process of sorting through experiences and memories to isolate and store the gist or specific detail of the memory. According to Harvard sleep researcher, Robert Stickgold, "When we dream, we get the pieces. When we wake, we can know the whole."

In Harold Boulette's article "Expanding Consciousness During Sleep", he writes:

It does make perfect sense that most of our spiritual awakening and consciousness expanding takes place while we sleep. A goldfish doesn't grow very big when kept in a small bowl. Consciousness can't expand much when trapped in the cage of conscious beliefs and thoughts. The mind has to be stilled and open to new things for expanding consciousness to happen.

As you can see, it is not necessarily "training" at all, but a re-learning of what is natural for each member of the family. Well-rested individuals spread calm centeredness instead of stressful anxiety to their children. Babies' innate schedule of development can then blossom without judgement, concern, or major interference.

How is Western Lifestyle Affecting Family Sleep?

Currently, many of us have little or no support within our immediate family unit. Although 68% of children live with two parents, there are more than 30% single parent households today compared to just 7% in 1950. There are 8.5 million single moms and 2.5 million single dads according to the U.S. Census Bureau. Some of these may have help in the form of nearby family members. Most of the support for single parents comes in the pre-natal period, although that is changing. Support is critical but getting less and less frequent and available in all areas of life, partly because of an aging population. For example, the family caregiver's ratio is a measure of the available family members who can take care of elderly parents. At one point not so long ago, that ratio was over seven to one, but soon it will be just three to one.

Separate from the issue of available support, is the issue of an over-stimulating environment. The amount of over-stimulation of the mind and information overload is staggering. It is estimated we make about 30,000 decisions a day. Wherever we look, there is competition for our attention. It trains our brains to be constantly vigilant but taxes our ability to be discerning about where to focus our attention, time and energy. This is draining, creating a mindset that is not conducive to rest and relaxation.

In an attempt to give us the energy we need for all our mental activity, many of us feed our bodies with processed foods high in sugar and rely on caffeine or energy drinks and supplements. These aids only provide a temporary solution and have the short-term effect of increasing arousal and energy. In the long term, they can deplete us, leave us feeling numb (if not exhausted), and the root of the problem remains unresolved.

Prescription medications are also on the rise. Prescription medications are usually given a lot of attention because of the increase in their use. For example, the prescription of antidepressants has increased 65% in the last twenty years. Medications for Attention Deficit Disorder (ADD) are also an issue.

According to the CDC's Morbidity and Mortality Weekly Report (MMWR),

> *The number of privately insured U.S. women ages 15-44 years who filled a prescription for a*

medicine to treat attention-deficit/hyperactivity disorder (ADHD) increased 344 percent between 2003 and 2015.

Even higher increases were reported for women in their late 20s and early 30s. For those ages 25-29 years, the number of women who filled a prescription for an ADHD medicine increased by 700 percent. The second largest increase was among women ages 30-34: a 560 percent increase.

While unquestionably there are times when medications of all sorts can be lifesaving and needed, prescribing seems to have gotten out of control as a superficial fix for a deeper-rooted issue that is most often overlooked. And usually, lifestyle or health solutions are not considered by your average medical practitioner who prescribes the medication. Furthermore, prescribing medications reinforces an approach that is based on looking for external, symptomatic fixes rather than more permanent internal solutions.

Now, while I support a holistic approach for just this reason, I should also say that there are many holistic practitioners out there that are so driven by prescribing herbs and supplements of all kinds: it's like everything is based on supplements, supplements and more supplements. We've got to be very careful about that because supplementation is just one part of the entire spectrum on the wheel of health. Our bodies are affected by our movements, emotions, sleep, nutrition, how we're structuring our lifestyle, and the rhythm and flow of our life. If we're just dependent on medicines or supplements, we're using symptomatic band-aids and not necessarily addressing the root of a problematic lifestyle. You can take all the supplements you want, but if you're food intake is deficient in nutrients, you have unresolved emotions or you are sedentary all the time, you're still limiting your optimal human function.

Obesity is on the rise due to a more sedentary lifestyle, as well as eating foods that are not nutrient dense. The answer is not getting supplements to manage your nutrient deficiency but eating foods that contain the nutrients our bodies need in the first place and that are conducive to sleep. This is important especially with infants and young children. Just because their daily caloric needs have been met and they are weighing in normal for their age, does not mean they are receiving all the nutrients their body needs. For example, I have worked with parents whose children have continuously woken up to feed - not out of habit or out of a sleep to feed association - but due to nutrient deficiencies.

Our body communicates to us in so many ways when it is out of balance. Aches, pain, exhaustion, hunger, mood are all clues to get to the root of the problem instead of bandaging the symptoms with quick fixes or medications.

Mar De Carlo

Parental Authority vs. Parental Leadership

In the world of parenting, quite often many of us play the authority role using power, coercion and making sure our children know who's the boss. This is how we learned, and believe, is the most effective way to parent. However, much research shows that authoritarian parenting limits children more than it benefits them. Indeed, most child sleep solutions require parents and caregivers to take on an authoritative role: giving orders and enforcing obedience, thus forcing the child to sleep according to the prescribed rules.

The definition of authority is the power or right to give orders, make decisions, and enforce obedience. Authority is a person or organization who has power, control or dominance in a particular political or administrative sphere. A lot of the sleep training solutions and sleep training mythologies are based on taking an authoritative role.

Now let's look at leadership and the leadership role. The definition of a leader or leadership is the action of leading a group of people or organization, guidance, direction, management, governance, and so on. It's very similar because they both pertain to words like power, but they're also very different.

At the same time, we want to be mindful of labels and how they impact our behavior, response and experience with our children. So, what helps is to reflect and question, essentially strengthen our consciousness.

For example:

When your child is experiencing sleep challenges, what comes up for you in handling the situation? Do you show up as an authority figure wanting to dominate, control and win over your child, or are you showing up as a leader coming from a place of understanding? Are you providing guidance, direction, holding the space, maintaining the boundaries, and coming off as a leader who isn't interested in force and coercion but teaching and role modeling?

It's not about "I win", or "they win", but it's about how you're going to guide them and how you set an example.

"I'm going to direct you with calm and confidence, I'm going to support you, navigate and lead, so that we can get from point A to point B."

That is more likely to lead to a beneficial outcome.

That's an important part of working with not only child sleep challenges, but all child challenges. It's about understanding the context, framing the problem and engaging your child in a collaborative effort to solve the problem. This is where we must be very honest with ourselves. It seems so much easier just to tell your kid what to do and force them to do it. However, force is the enemy of engagement. The more you force your child, the more resistant they are likely to be. And if they do accept being forced, it's likely to have a negative effect on their self-esteem, as they see that other people control their lives. Moreover, any problem is an opportunity for a child to learn the critical life skill of adaptation and an opportunity for us to learn about our own limitations. You rob them and yourself of that opportunity if you make the decision and force behavior on them.

Let's look at the following case example of a five-year-old girl, Hannah who is the oldest of three children, with two younger brothers. She has her own room and sleeps in her own bed, but about five months ago, she wanted to sleep in her brothers' room, due to being scared. Hannah needs her mom and dad to sit in the room at the start of bedtime every night. Once she falls asleep (which takes about 20 -30 minutes), she will wake about 2.5 - 3 hours later and walk into mom and dad's room. Mom or dad walk her immediately back but she cries unless mom or dad sit back in a chair in her room so she can fall asleep. Mom typically sits down on her bed until she is asleep. From there, Hannah will wake a few hours later and will quietly sneak into mom and dad's bed to sleep for the rest of the night. When I surveyed parents and sleep professionals and asked them what they think the root cause of Hannah's sleep challenge is, the average response was that Hannah has a boundary issue. They felt that by treating her behavior as a boundary issue and implementing sleep training, Hannah would remember how to sleep independently. Investigating and addressing Hannah's fear was not a consideration although, Hannah's fear is the root issue of her sleep challenge. By not addressing Hannah's fear, she is taught to suppress her emotion in order to abide her parent's sleep rules. When you approach your child's behavior, like in Hannah's case, from an authoritative perspective, it's easy to mistake his or her sleep behavior as a boundary issue but, when you approach your child's behavior from a leadership perspective, you guide your child to process the emotion preventing him or her from sleeping.

Intermittent Reinforcement

Intermittent reinforcement is a commonly used term in the world of child sleep and parenting in general.

Intermittent reinforcement is when rules, rewards or personal boundaries are handed out or enforced inconsistently and occasionally, which usually encourages another person to keep pushing until they get what they want from you without changing their own behavior.

I often encounter parents and sleep professionals who fear intermittent reinforcement and want to avoid it.

What I see happening most often is that parents and professionals take intermittent reinforcement out of context and apply it to situations and circumstances that developmentally or physically do not make sense for a child's behavior especially when it comes to sleep.

For example, if my child is having an issue with wetting their pants and it is related to a medical issue, trying to enforce a reward/punishment or rule around it is not logical because the root of the child's wetting their pants is something currently beyond their control that needs assistance.

If my child, who sleeps independently and no longer co-sleeps with me, experiences a nightmare and wants to jump into bed with me one night, I am not going to fear intermittent reinforcement. I do not want my children to fear or ever feel that I cannot be available to them under such circumstances.

If my eight-month-old child is under the weather and is waking up at night needing my attention because of the discomfort they are going through, it does not make sense to be afraid of intermittent reinforcement if I respond to them.

If my child is going through a gradual night weaning process, I am going to put my energy and focus in encouraging and supplementing their feeding needs during the day and not fear if they still need a feed here and there at night during this process. Because as the saying goes,

"Energy flows where attention goes." ~ Michael Beckwith

Of course, it is important that we are a role model to our children on how to honor agreements, rules and boundaries. However, if we look at the definition of reinforcement, it is "the process of encouraging or establishing a belief or pattern of behavior, especially by encouragement or reward.

Human evolution involves expansion, which means that as we develop and mature, we don't get stuck in beliefs or patterns, but free ourselves of them.

In modern civilization, a child's natural sleep developmental patterns are often perceived as an inconvenience to the structure, schedule, and stressed lifestyle of modern-day living. As a result, many families resort to sleep training and reinforcement in order to get their child's body to conform with modern lifestyle, structure and beliefs.

Since sleep is fundamental for survival and a natural recurring state of mind and body, the human body does not need reinforcement to sleep just like we do not need reinforcement to breathe. Therefore, sleep does not need to be taught or trained. It's a matter of being conscious, the of root cause of a sleep challenge and addressing the things that are interfering with the body's natural rhythms, homeostasis and inviting a lifestyle for the whole family that supports sleep.

Taking a Team Approach

Another issue or concern I hear often is the fear of being an overly involved parent.

You may be thinking, "If I attend too much to my child, I'm going to create a co-dependency leading to a negative sleep association." Then that fear comes up, right? And then as a result of having that fear, the fear begins to mold and shape our perception and reality.

This may also lead a parent to think, "Well, my child has to learn to be independent. I need to let them figure challenges out on their own. Therefore, I'm going to give them more space and let them cry it out."
When this happens, a child may learn to sleep on his or her own, but at the cost of the limiting perspective that they live in a world where they need to handle things on their own without the support of their loved one.

An alternative is to take a team approach by meeting your child's needs, offering them the space they need to process and learn, while at the same time providing them with security, safety, and your presence.

What makes a team strong is that everybody in that team is taken into consideration. Everybody in that team plays a role. Everybody in that team is giving to and receiving from one another. It's not about teaching one another to fend for themselves. We want to be aware of our whole family dynamic and understand what everybody's needs are and how we can be supportive so we can all grow individually and together.

When we look at child sleep, we want to look at our family's sleep and wake cycles, because they all matter. They all affect each other as we co-exist as a family living together.

The Role of Crying

"Not only can a newborn not distinguish between his senses, he also is unable to make a distinction between sensations that originate within his own body and those that come from outside of it. As far as he is concerned, the outside world and his body are one and the same. What happens outside, happens inside his body too."

Excerpt from *Why They Cry*, (Hetty van de Rijt and Frans Plooij, 1996)

Crying and child sleep is a hot and very sensitive topic. Often you will find parents and professionals in heated discussions for or against crying when faced with child sleep challenges they want to resolve.

But what is very interesting, is that getting to the root of why a child is crying or wants to cry is usually not at the forefront of investigation or discussion.

Crying plays a very important role in communication and the release of frustration and emotion.

When people say "no-cry solution", that automatically becomes a behavior methodology. This means they are trying to control a situation of no-crying behavior in order to support a child sleeping.

In the same fashion, a "cry it out" solution also becomes a behavior methodology because we are also trying to control a child by ignoring their cry in order to get them to sleep.

Usually, the two styles of parental responses to child crying that I witness are:

A fear or discomfort of one's child crying where the immediate reaction is to shush or stop the crying. This unintentionally sends a message to a child that crying is not an acceptable behavior.

A frustration or discomfort of one's child crying where the immediate reaction is to ignore the child's crying behavior. This also unintentionally sends a message to a child that crying is not an acceptable behavior.

Yet these two styles of parental responses are at odds with one another.

When our child is learning how to crawl or walk, obviously as parents and caregivers, we're going to monitor the situation. We want to make sure the child is going to be safe. We're going to be helping them along the way, but we're not going to do the job for them, right? We're not going to try to force them to roll or crawl or walk a certain way. We're going to be there and hold the space for them as they learn to do it. Then we get excited. "Oh! Look! Look! They finally sat up!" "Oh! Look! They're standing and they're holding it!" Right?

It's the same thing when it comes to emotion. To stop a child from crying or to just allow them to excessively cry is unnatural. It's almost like forcing a child to not take another step in their process of learning how to walk.

There's a big difference between the two opposites. While we're saying that we don't want to suppress a child's natural response to cry, we also don't want to ignore a cry and force a situation that is that is going to lead the child to crying more unnaturally.

Crying, in and of itself, is not a problem. In my opinion, this is one of the biggest mistakes I feel that's happening out there in the world of child sleep and one of the motivating drives behind my Holistic Science of Sleep Method.

Crying should not be the main focal point of any sleep solution but rather a signal to inform us of what our child is trying to communicate so that we may get to the root of their behavior and discover the most appropriate solution.

If a child will naturally cry in a situation, we want to invite that while evaluating the reasoning behind their cry. At the same time, we also want to be mindful of an excessive cry or suppressed cry.

There is a fine line between methodologies that offer minimal crying and no-cry solutions. Their aim is to ease, soothe and gently transition a child so that the child's response is not drastically impacted by the change in sleep situation.

I believe that the intention of these methodologies is to introduce gentler ways of working with a child. But the problem with any of those solutions, is that we're trying to control a behavior. Behavior is a response to internal and external stimuli; we want to address the root of the behavior, not control it.

The behavior will naturally change once we address the underlying problem and apply a solution to it. Once we uncover what the root of the problem is, or the situation is, and we know how to then apply a solution to it, the behavior will naturally change.

But what's happening, is people are jumping toward the behavior first to find a solution and working backwards from there.

Every child is different, and their response will be different depending on many factors. Every human being is different. We all have different lifestyle, habits, temperaments, personalities and expressions that are continuously evolving and changing.

As a result, my Holistic Science of Sleep Method approach deals with a crying child by first accepting and embracing it. Not ignoring the child and letting them cry or trying to stop their cries, but accepting the crying. Accept that they are crying, and through this acceptance, give yourself an opportunity to be present for your child, listen and discover what is needed for him or her in that moment.

If feelings of discomfort, frustration or judgement arise within you from their crying that is something for you to face and work on, not your child. Children are such great teachers and often uncover unresolved aspects of ourselves.

Many of us may not be conscious of or are not taking responsibility for our own behaviors and reactions that we model for our children. That can and usually does exacerbate the way they are feeling.

Since birth, children learn and respond to signals from their parents and other people in their environment about which emotions and actions are appropriate in a certain context or situation. Infants observe the behavior of others and imitate their actions and behaviors. This psychology is referred to as "social referencing".

"Feel what you need to feel and then let it go, do not let it consume you." ~ Dhiman

The emotions we feel affect our children and shape their development and perspective of the world. It is important and normal to show our children a full spectrum of emotions but more importantly model for them how to healthfully and safely deal with them.

It may feel challenging at first because many of us have feelings, judgements and our own experiences with crying that can get in the way of how we respond to another's cry. We also have been trained and formed habits of how we react to crying. But in every challenge lies an opportunity and our children give us an opportunity to strengthen our consciousness, understand how to deal with our own discomforts, judgements and feelings that in turn will support their development and growth.

If we allow our children to feel their feelings in our safe, nonjudgmental presence and we model how to feel and move through our emotions, they will learn to do the same. We want them to know that we're there for them every step of the way. We want to make sure we're meeting their needs.

There are so many reasons a child could be crying, but what I commonly see are assumptions being made. Before one even has the chance to get to the root of why a child is crying, a method is already being implemented.

Often, I have worked with cases, similar to the one my graduate experienced, shared in my Holistic Science of Sleep Method Chapter, where a child is waking up multiple times a night, and the assumption is that they have simply not learned how to sleep. The parents go to their pediatrician who may advise them to let the baby "cry it out", or they go to a sleep consultant who may take a gentler approach. But the whole picture is not evaluated, and the root cause remains undiscovered.

Children may be waking up at night for several reasons that have nothing to do with what the parent or expert may be assuming. Therefore, it is important to evaluate all the areas in that child's life that may be influencing their sleep beyond the commonly assumed ones.

The Power & Influence of Nutrition for Sleep

Most child sleep books, sleep consultants and doctors do not bring enough attention to how nutrition plays a crucial role in pregnancy, child and adult sleep. By far, it is an underestimated, underlying cause for many sleep challenges.

Nutritional Deficiencies

According to Dr. Mercola, factors contributing to poor sleep include vitamin and mineral deficiencies.

Magnesium deficiency can cause insomnia; lack of potassium can lead to difficulty staying asleep; and vitamin D deficiency has been linked to excessive daytime sleepiness.

Iron

In addition, iron deficiency has also been linked to sleep issues. In the following article, *"Magnesium and Iron: The 'Silver Bullet' Solutions to Better Baby Sleep?"* writer Emily DeJeu shares:

Low levels of iron have also been linked to sleep issues. A 2010 study indicates that IDA (iron deficiency anemia) in infants can cause altered brain patterns that lead to disrupted sleep. IDA has also been linked to RLS (restless leg syndrome) and sleep apnea, two conditions known to cause insomnia. All of this research suggests that having healthy levels of iron in the bloodstream contributes to deeper, more restorative sleep for both children and adults.

According to John Hopkins Medicine:

In the last 20 years, there has been a substantial amount of research into understanding the cause of RLS. From that research there appears to be three factors which are pertinent to the disease: brain concentrations of iron, brain dopamine concentrations and genes.

The single most consistent finding and the strongest environmental risk factor associated with RLS is iron insufficiency. Professor Nordlander first recognized the association between iron deficiency and RLS and reported that treatment of the iron deficiency markedly improved, if not eliminated, the RLS symptoms.

DHA

Another example is the correlation between child sleep and DHA deficiency.

In Dr. David Perlmutter's article, "DHA Improves Sleep in Children", he writes:

British researchers publishing in the Journal of Sleep Research evaluated the sleep patterns of 395 children aged 7-9 years. In addition, they performed a blood analysis on these children to measure their levels of DHA, an omega-3 fatty acid.

As had been reported in earlier studies, the number of children having trouble with sleep was a remarkable 40%. When the researchers looked specifically at the measurements of total nightly sleep, they discovered a correlation with blood

DHA levels. Lower levels of DHA correlated with a reduction in the length of time children were sleeping while higher blood DHA levels were associated with significantly better sleep.

The study revealed that those children getting the DHA showed not only better quality of sleep, but significantly fewer and shorter night-wakings and an increase in sleep duration by an impressive 58 minutes, when compared to the children receiving the placebo.

In normal sleep, there is an increase in the hormone leptin that turns off appetite. However, with disturbed or delayed sleep, the opposite occurs: there's an increase in the hormone ghrelin that turns on appetite. Going down to the kitchen for a snack at midnight isn't just because you're frustrated about insomnia, hormones can also be driving your appetite.

Melatonin is one of the most important hormones to help you optimize your sleep, as it plays a crucial role in your circadian rhythm or internal clock.

Anti and Pro-sleep Foods

Most of my clients and surprisingly child sleep consultants I have worked with have not been aware of anti and pro-sleep foods and their influences and effects on sleep.

Eating habits also influence your ability to relax and fall asleep. Eating habits can include things like the pace at which you eat, how mindful or mindless you are when you are eating, the kinds of foods you consistently eat, eating when you are not hungry, etc.

The food we eat can severely affect our sleep and set off a cascade of negative reactions that can lead to a wellness and sleep downward spiral. This applies to all of us at any age.

Of course, there are certain foods and substances that can influence the wake/sleep cycle. Caffeine in particular can keep you awake. And remember, caffeine is not just in coffee and tea, it's in chocolate and hidden in many popular Starbucks drinks, too. When you're having that chocolate snack watching TV at night, don't forget that it will likely delay your sleep onset. The general rule for a good sleep routine is no caffeine after 2pm.

The brain and the gut are intimately connected, and it should be no surprise that what happens in the stomach and intestines affects sleep. Remember, food is not just – or even – about calories. Food provides the building blocks of your entire brain and body that keep our body functioning well or lead it to spin out of control.

It is also important to remember that the food you eat during pregnancy is shaping your baby's environment and potentially having major effects on its development. And if your pregnancy eating habits are contributing to your poor sleep, that too, is potentially affecting your baby's development. The same dynamic applies to breast feeding. Your food choices are going to affect your baby, for better or for worse.

Here are some foods to avoid most of the time, if not completely, but certainly later in the day.

Trans fat in the forms of vegetable-based oils like safflower, canola, palm and similar oils can all create an inflammatory response. They contain toxins, which increases the risk of inflammation. As a result, these oils and types of foods increase the stress hormone cortisol. In the normal state, the body shuts down cortisol production as night approaches to relax the body. However, that process can be reversed with trans-fat oils, making it difficult to get to sleep and stay asleep. Reduced cortisol is a necessary part of the relaxation and sleep induction process.

High sugar foods increase glucose levels, insulin and increase cortisol. So, be careful about a big sugar fix from candy too late in the day. Especially be careful of so-called "health foods" like juices and fat free foods that have massive amounts of sugar, like some fruit juices and even some yogurts. Watch out for fat free foods, like some yogurts, that compensate for the lack of fat by adding massive amounts of sugar.

Alcohol can be something of a paradox. Because it makes most people relaxed and sleepy, it is assumed that it therefore is good for sleep. Typically, people drink it in the evening in order to relax and wind down. While alcohol does indeed help you get off to sleep, it negatively effects later stages of sleep, like dreaming and deep sleep, which are critical parts of the healing and recharging process. So, while alcohol might get you to sleep initially, it will also lead to a disrupted and unfulfilled night's rest.

Low-fiber Carbs, such as processed foods, snack foods and sugary drinks, have the worst of two worlds. They contain sugar and not much fiber which would help slow the absorption process. Without that fiber, these foods and the sugar contained in them gets quickly absorbed, leading to a spike in blood-glucose levels, insulin, and, you guessed it, cortisol.

Low-quality Meats come from those animals typically raised with poor-quality nutrition, added hormones and antibiotics. These constituents lead to meat that has an excess of omega-6 fatty acids. While omega-3 fatty acid combats inflammation, omega-6 increases it, once again increasing cortisol. Foods from animals raised in a natural and sustainable way are much healthier, with a better balance of the omega fatty acids.

The timing of eating, the food eaten, and combining of foods have a big impact on sleep. Digesting food requires more energy than any other function in the human body.

Avoid heavy meals for at least two to three hours prior to sleep. Not only does the process of indigestion interfere with sleep, it can create a lot of discomfort. In addition, the natural drive for food shuts down as the evening wears on, which is a good thing as it reduces hunger. But if you are still processing and metabolizing food from a late dinner, the hunger inhibiting process can not only be delayed but reversed. The digestive process is an active one, not compatible with sleeping, regardless of what you have been eating.

In some cases, cortisol and the appetite suppressing hormone are not turned off, which can lead to late night snacking of high sugar foods – a very dangerous behavior that not only significantly disrupts sleep, but can easily lead to rapid weight gain, and all the consequences thereof.

Anti-Inflammatory Nutrition & Lifestyle to Support Sleep

Inflammation may be a key factor which is limiting your body from quality sleep. Reducing inflammation will not only improve your sleep, but your overall health. In addition, improving your sleep will reduce inflammation.

Examples of foods that cause inflammation:

- Sugar and High Fructose Corn Syrup
- Saturated Fats
- Trans Fats
- Omega 6 Fatty Acids-Vegetable and Seed Oils
- Refined Carbohydrates
- MSG
- Gluten and Casein
- Alcohol
- Processed Meat

Examples of Anti-Inflammatory Foods:

- Fruits

- o Veggies
- o Fatty Fish
- o Avocados
- o Almonds
- o Turmeric
- o Extra Virgin Olive Oil

While nutrition plays a key role to reducing inflammation, living a minimal stress and active lifestyle is important as well.

Food Sensitivities and Sleep

I have worked with many clients and professionals whose child sleep challenge cases were due to food sensitivities.

Whereas food allergies are easier to detect due to the immediate reaction one has to food, food sensitivities are usually a bit more challenging to uncover because it can take up to 72 hours for symptoms to display themselves and symptoms also vary.

For example, symptoms can include:

- o Skin irritations or rashes
- o Stomach pains
- o Gas
- o Indigestion
- o Behavioral issues
- o Fatigue
- o Frequent infections

Some of the common food sensitivity culprits:

- o Gluten
- o Dairy
- o Soy
- o Eggs
- o Nuts
- o Shellfish
- o Peanuts

If you have a history of food sensitivities, allergies, or suspect your child does, it is important to have the situation evaluated by a qualified professional.

Colic/Fussy Babies

While not every colic case may be due to diet, a good majority of them are, so it helps to rule out any possible dietary causes. Despite denial that colic has any correlation to gastrointestinal problems or the breastfeeding mother's diet, many families' colic problems were solved by changing their diet.

For example, from a book review on colic, one parent shares:

> *My baby was clearly hurting, and her cries told me so. Experimentation has led me to conclude that both my diet (which now excludes dairy) as well as acid reflux were overlapping issues causing her pain. By trying a new diet, we saw improvement with gas problems first and then later solved the acid problems with reflux medication. My pediatrician supported my instincts and now we have a much happier baby. She still fusses a little but no longer cries from pain.*

Some babies are just fussy, and some are trying to tell you something. I'm glad I listened.

Research also backs up the correlation between diet and colic.

According to WebMD.com's article, "Mom's Diet May Be Key to Cutting Baby's Colic":

> *A study published in the current issue of Pediatrics suggests that excluding highly allergenic foods from a nursing mother's diet could reduce crying and fussiness in her newborn's first six weeks of life.*
>
> *The study involved 90 breastfeeding mothers whose infants showed significant signs of colic. Breastfeeding-only infants with colic who were less than 6 weeks of age were asked to participate.*
>
> *For the 10-day study, about half of the mothers avoided eggs, cow's milk, peanuts, tree nuts, wheat, soy and fish; the other half continued to eat those foods for a week. The mothers first recorded*

how often their babies cried or fussed on days one and two of the study. Then each group of mothers started its diet regimens for a week. The mothers recorded their babies' crying and fussing again on days eight and nine.

At the end of the study, 74% of infants in the low-allergen group experienced at least a 25% reduction in crying and fussing. Only 37% of infants in the standard-diet group had a similar reduction. "These findings suggest that maternal intake of food allergens is an important factor in the [development] of infantile colic among breastfed infants," the researchers write.

The researchers caution that breastfeeding mothers should not make drastic diet changes on their own. "Elimination diets have associated risks, particularly if sustained for long periods," they write. "The nutritional progress of the infant and the mother needs to be monitored closely by an experienced dietitian."

Dehydration

Dehydration is more common in adults and children than most people are aware of and it can affect the quality of sleep.

According to the National Sleep Foundation:

> *Hydration also plays a critical role in how well (or not) you sleep at night. Understanding the impact of your daily fluid intake on your nighttime slumber will go a long way to improving the quality of your sleep. Going to bed even mildly dehydrated can disrupt your sleep. Surprised? Dehydration causes your mouth and nasal passages to become dry, setting you up for sleep-disruptive snoring and a parched throat and hoarseness in the morning.*

> *A lack of pre-bed fluids can also lead to nocturnal leg cramps that may keep you awake. In addition to the frustration of fragmented sleep, being dehydrated during night can compromise your*

alertness, energy, and cognitive performance the following day.

They recommend:

Focus on drinking plenty of non-caffeinated fluids regularly throughout the day. Women need approximately 91 ounces daily from beverages and foods, while men should aim for about 125 ounces. Waiting until bedtime to do your drinking sets you up for multiple nighttime bathroom trips (if this happens frequently to you, it may be a condition called nocturia) making it difficult to achieve quality sleep and making it tougher to wake up in the morning. Practice spreading your fluid intake throughout your day to maximize the odds of sleeping soundly at night.

With children, it is important to monitor and be aware of signs or factors that can put them at a higher risk for dehydration.

For example, some high-risk factors may include:

- o Fever
- o Excessive Sweating
- o Hot Temperatures
- o Illness
- o Vomiting
- o Diarrhea

Dehydration signs include and not limited to:

- o Dark Colored Urine
- o Little or No Urine
- o Dry or Cold skin
- o Sunken Eyes
- o Low Energy Levels
- o No Tears When Crying
- o Dry or Cracked Lips

The Case for Real Food

When one realizes the fact that the vast majority of processed commercial food negatively impacts sleep quality, and that diet is often the major factor in sleep imbalances, the initial reaction from some is to feel limited and restricted as to what they can now eat. This, of course, is really nothing but a misperception, because the fact is that there is an incredible bounty of natural foods available to humans nowadays, like no other time in history. The variety of natural foods (like fruits and vegetables) that humans had access to 50 or 100 years ago is only a fraction compared to what we have now. Modern transportation has opened up the farms of the world and brought this incredible earth bounty to our local markets and to our tables for us and our children to enjoy.

Next time you feel limited in your food choices, consider this fact alone: There are approximately one to two thousand species of fruits to choose from, and many of these species of fruits have thousands of varieties within their species. That means there are actually millions of different types of fruits to enjoy.

There are roughly 5000 varieties of apples, 1600 varieties of bananas, 500 varieties of avocados, and 10,000 varieties of grapes, to name a few. Also consider the fact that there are roughly 20,000-300,000 species of edible plants on the planet. Consumers all over the world now have access to tropical fruits from all sorts of locations. Just a few decades ago, many of these fruits were not available to consumers anywhere, except where they were grown locally. The variety of healthy natural foods available to us are increasing daily, so much so that it is almost impossible to keep up with. You could eat a different fruit every day for the rest of your life and still not taste all the fruits available on the planet.

When we move our attention from what we can't have to what we can have, our options for healthy food choices become abundant.

A healthy balanced body with a healthy appetite craves foods that are natural to our diet. However, many of us have become so psychologically conditioned with our relationship to food. As a result, we do not eat in response to actual hunger, but in response to many other things; for example, to an emotion or to a strategy we heard works best. We then develop an imbalance and disconnection with our body and its relationship to food. When the body has certain addictions and a distorted appetite, it typically requires heavily stimulating and heavily seasoned foods just to be appealing. A person with a strong, healthy appetite finds unprocessed natural foods, such as fruits and certain greens, to be highly appealing and delicious. One doesn't require salty/sweet/acidic/fatty enhancements with every bite, nor do they require foods full of stimulants or addictive substances to enjoy their food.

The Importance of Gradual Transition

Another big sleep issue is the critical importance of how we transition from day to night and night to day. The lifestyle in our modern-day culture makes it easy to carry the day into the night, even after the sun sets, and easy to wake up abruptly with our alarm clocks.

During the night, our body still thinks it is daytime because our environments mimic it. For example, exposure to shining bright lights, screens and noise after the sun sets is very common.

If we look at nature, when the sun starts to set, of course we're going to hear frogs and other animals, crickets and different creatures out there, but the tone of the sounds is much quieter. It's almost like a blanket of silence: it's a very easeful tone that exists where in the daytime there's a louder buzz out there in nature. What's happening is that we're filling up our days and we're going from activity to activity, many of us over-stimulated, and we don't have any time to pause, no time to slow down. The sun sets, but we keep going. As a result, the mind and the body don't get to experience a transition from day to night and that absolutely affects sleep.

During the day, the average person trains themselves to get jolted awake in order to start their day and do not allow for a gradual transition from night to day.

In a news story covered by ABC News:

> *True, natural light is better to wake up to than an alarm clock. According to Research by the National Institute of Industrial Health in Japan, despite the popularity of using an alarm clock, waking up to a jolting noise can be bad for your heart. Waking up abruptly can cause higher blood pressure and heart rate.*

Artificial Light

Indeed, one of the major sources of these differences is the widespread availability of artificial light, which has led to significant changes in sleep patterns in the Industrial West since its introduction in the mid-19th century. Today we sleep at least one hour less each night than was the custom even a century ago and probably several hours less than before industrialization and electricity. According to some studies, artificial lighting has encouraged both later sleep onset times and the tendency to sleep in a single concentrated burst through the night. This monophasic sleep is more segmented, compared to broken up sleep patterns -- polyphasic or biphasic sleep -- still found in many underdeveloped or nomadic societies.

Dr. Thomas A. Wehr conducted a study in 1992 to gain some insight into natural sleep patterns prior to the use of excessive nighttime illumination. He found that when healthy adults were prohibited from using artificial light at night from dusk until dawn, their sleep patterns went through an unusual transformation. Sleep became biphasic with two stages of 3-5 hours of sleep separated by 1-3 hour waking period. (In Short Photoperiods, Human Sleep Is Biphasic: Journal of Sleep Research 1(2):103-107 · June 1992)

I'm not suggesting that we go back in time and we avoid or ignore or restrict ourselves from modern day industrialization. We want to welcome in the advances of today's society, of electricity and our lifestyles, in a way that complements and integrates natural patterns more effectively and beneficially to sleep.

The Power of Sunlight

Over the years, I have witnessed an increasing amount of concern over sun exposure due to ozone depletion, global warming, and skin cancer along with an increase in sunscreen usage and warnings that to deal with this concern. Likewise, in the last few years, there has been a huge increase in the studies showing the health benefits of sunshine. Sun exposure has now been shown to prevent literally dozens of major illnesses including cancer. There is no question that too much of anything, even something that is essential and good for you, can become a problem. Clearly one can overdose on vitamins, herbs, drugs, and even water. Too much of just about anything can become toxic in the body. It's the same with our good friend the sun. Sunshine has tremendous health benefits and many scientists have been finding through their research that exposure to sunshine as little as 15 minutes a day 3 times per week has been shown to ward of all sorts of illness and disease, and greatly affect the mood of those battling depression. Sunshine also regulates and balances hormone levels and circadian rhythms so those with sleep issues can also benefit from more sun exposure.

According to a study discussed in Scientific American, "Vitamin D deficiency soars in the U.S.", as three-quarters of U.S. teens and adults are now deficient in vitamin D, the so-called "sunshine vitamin".

Seven out of ten U.S. children have low levels of vitamin D according to a study of over 6,000 children by researchers at Albert Einstein College of Medicine of Yeshiva University.

Melatonin, as mentioned previously, is one of the most important hormones necessary in order to optimize sleep but sun exposure just as equally plays an important role.

In John Douillard's article, "How Sun Exposure Affects Sleep and Melatonin Production" he writes:

> *Melatonin is a hormone produced by the pineal gland, and it is MUCH more than just a sleep hormone.*

> *Like the janitor who comes in at night to clean the floors and wash the windows, melatonin is the*

body's most powerful detoxification and rejuvenation agent.

While the role melatonin plays in our health is still not fully understood, studies suggest that without a good dose of daily sun exposure, we do not produce optimal levels of melatonin. Sadly, modern humans are getting too much light at night and not bright enough light during the day.

If you are looking for a better night's sleep, or to boost the benefits of melatonin as an anti-aging hormone and detoxifying hormone, the amount of sunlight you get during the day is as critical as the amount of darkness you get at night.

Most people with sleep imbalances put a lot of energy into eye masks or shades that completely block out any ambient light from their bedroom, but they may not be putting the same amount of attention towards getting the daily sunlight they need to produce optimal melatonin levels.

Imagine how this affects our children.

How many children are not only exposed to bright lights but screens right before bed and then expected to fall right asleep?

How many children must be woken up by alarm clock to get to school on time? Which raises another interesting issue about our many school systems and their expected start times in a modern society that encourages daytime activity and light exposure at night.

How many children get proper sunlight exposure with today's overriding fear of the sun?

As a result, a holistic perspective and approach supports the integration and development of healthy lifestyles very necessary in today's society.

People not only need to be more educated about sleep in general and how their health and lifestyle patterns interact with, and are affected by their sleep, but they also need to understand how to practically implement healthy habits into their lifestyle that supports sleep.

These lifestyle components include gradual lifestyle changes, not overnight or extreme changes. A core principle is honoring the value and the necessity of sleep. In some ways, sleep has gotten a bad rap. It's as if sleep is for those who don't have enough drive or ambition to work into the late hours. Or they consider themselves weak because they don't stay up all night to finish that project. That is a huge mistake. Sleep can't be disregarded. It can take several days, if not weeks, to make up for one very poor night's sleep. It's not as if I can finally sleep in a couple of days when I have finished this project.

Sure, there are going to be moments when someone will be up, have very little sleep for a few nights, or a period of time, due to special circumstances. However, that's very different from someone who disregards sleep and their body's need for it. Surrendering to sleep is as important as sleep and wake-up times. We need to honor and adapt co-regulating rhythms, energetic qualities, and allow for any new transitions. We can't minimize sleep!

Most people are not aware that between 10:00 p.m. and 2:00 a.m. is the most optimal time for the body to naturally physically repair itself. From 2:00 a.m. to 6:00 a.m. is the most optimal and natural time for the psychological repair. There's also a period of time throughout the day, throughout a 24-hour period, where our organs also are most optimally repaired. A lot of times I look at those factors and weigh them in both child and adult sleep. When looking at an infant or a newborn, it's important to recognize that their 24-hour sleep and wake times have shorter windows which eventually will increase in length.

I'm often looking for signs and signals of any kind that might be inhibiting my clients' natural rhythm of sleep time and wake times. I have found that often parents and professionals underestimate how much internal and external influences affect sleep. For example, a baby may have a food sensitivity, be on a medication or they might have recently been vaccinated. If a baby is going through a growth spurt, teething, sick, changing formulas, or a change in breastfeeding, then all of these factors can interrupt and inhibit the rhythm and natural flow of wake and sleep cycles.

However, there have been many times I have encountered sleep consultants and families who are so rigid with following timed charts of exact sleep and wake windows that in doing so, add additional stress to themselves. They may also miss other influences affecting the natural rhythm of sleep and wake times for their child.

As a result, it is beneficial to build a keen sense of awareness observing our children and their reactions to the various internal and external influences that may be inhibiting their sleep.

Routine, Consistency &
Stress Management

There has been a lot written recently about sleep hygiene. These books and articles recognize the influence of certain behaviors on the process of getting to sleep and staying asleep. It's important that we understand these tools and their value not just for our own sleep, but for the increase in mindfulness it will give us about child sleep, too. The same principles apply.

Routine and Consistency

The body loves consistency, rhythms, regularity and stability within a flexible range. So many factors and systems are involved in the wake/sleep cycle that the more normalized it becomes, the better. It doesn't help if one part of your body is trying to get to sleep, while another part is signaling it to be awake, which is what can easily happen.

A routine does not need to be rigid; it just needs to be regular. If 80% of the time your body is consistent and regular with a certain way and time of eating, a time for sleeping, and so on, you'll be in a stable rhythm. The 15% or 20% of the time it's not in rhythm will not be a big deal.

Regular and normalized sleep and wake-up times are important in establishing synchronized rhythms that will help your sleep. One of the problems for school-age children is that they have one rhythm for school days and a completely different one for non-school days. Given that children are in school about 50% of the time, they often have two very different sleep routines. And switching between them can be challenging and take much longer than most people assume.

It's not only the timing of falling asleep and waking up that needs to be normalized, it's the routines that accompany the preparation for sleep. These routines should involve a scaling down of stimulation that would otherwise keep you awake.

Lighting, as mentioned earlier, is one of the keys to effective sleep preparation. Our bodies respond to illumination which determines either the maintenance, increase or decrease in wakefulness. So, illumination should be minimal in the sleep preparation phase, and absent during sleep. There is a reason why a full moon is associated with more activity in the animal kingdom.

This also addresses the issue of televisions, and screens in general, in the bedroom. Ideally, a bedroom is a place for peace, rest, sleep and intimacy. It's not a movie theater. When you turn on the TV, iPad or smartphone, you're inviting the rest of the world into this sacred space. You're also tuning your brain to the outside world, which increases attention and alertness.

When the wind-down towards sleep is more internally focused, this will reduce levels of energy and arousal. Reading a book or doing some simple puzzles (in low illumination) allow for energy to be downregulated, setting the scene for an easy, gradual transition to sleep.

Stress management is also a major consideration for parents in the post-partum phase, especially during fourth trimester. And becoming aware of our breathing pattern is an important key. Our breathing pattern is an indicator that alerts us to the physical and mental state we are in. We can use our breathing pattern as a way of managing tension and recalibrating our nervous system.

A lot of times parents are unaware of their breathing patterns. They're unaware that they're breathing through their mouth. They're unaware they are holding their breath. They're unaware that their breath is shallow or quick. So, I usually have my clients evaluate their breath with a breath check-in. This is one of the tools I provide families during pregnancy and the fourth trimester. For example, I tell them: Notice your breath. Then I ask questions like: Do you feel yourself breathing heavy and fast and shallow? Do you feel yourself breathing only in through your mouth, for example? And when my clients catch themselves doing that, I teach proper breathing mechanics and encourage them to stop for a moment, take a pause and realign with optimal breathing. Just being more aware of their body, closing their mouth, slowing down their breathing a little bit, and inviting a calmer energy begins an instant transformation.

Ideally, you don't want to go to sleep frustrated, angry and generally stressed. One of the major stress chemicals, cortisol, is naturally reduced as the day wears on and is pivotal in falling asleep. However, when stressed, that cortisol will continue to flow through you, keeping you very alert and even disrupting other hormonal changes (like an increase in leptin turning off appetite) so you not only feel more stressed but also hungrier, too.

Many times, when I work with families and they hear the words, "lifestyle change" they think "Oh gosh, I've got to start eating carrots and celery sticks and salads." Or "I've got to start taking one-hour yoga classes and join the gym." but, no, you don't have to initially make immediate big changes. It's the little baby steps that lead to the big steps and often these steps can be integrated very easily into one's daily rhythm and flow. It's small things that make a big difference. For example, you can start out with a small baby step of taking a three-to-five-minute pause, two to three times a day after breakfast, lunch or dinner or after you've put your baby down to nap. There are so many great options and techniques to choose from. I meet my clients where they are at, guide them to turn inward, find out what feels most suitable for them and then work on a practical and achievable plan to implement it.

In this respect, I also use technology like the CALM app. You can get it on any smart phone, android, iPhone, etc. There are many other similar apps, too. The CALM app is practical because you can also use it in airplane mode, so you don't have to worry about wi-fi and you can select the scenery that you want. You can set a scene of a beach, mountain side, or waterfall to get you out of the moment of stress and take a pause. You also can do unguided or guided meditations. The guided meditations go from simple breathing to a body scan, and yes, there's one for sleep and for different brain states: Deep sleep, calming, anxiety, deep concentration, emergency calm for immediate relief. What's really cool about it is you can select durations of 3 minutes, 5 minutes or 10 minutes.

Once you have gone through a guided meditation with the CALM app, you would take notice of your mental state and how you feel. That is one of many ways to be able to reset, recharge your body and be more prepared to then handle and face your family dynamics with a newborn.

I also highly recommend Yoga Nidra to my clients. As I mentioned in my "Pregnancy sleep tips", according to Guru Swami Satyananda, one hour of Yoga Nidra is believed to equal four hours of quality sleep.

"Live classes are available in Yoga Nidra, as well as apps, audio guides, and a modern-day version of Yoga Nidra called "iRest".

iRest is a meditation practice that can be done in a class setting or on one's own, based on the ancient tradition of Yoga Nidra, and adapted to suit the conditions of modern life. When practiced regularly - a little and often - iRest enables you to meet each moment of your life with unshakable peace and wellbeing, no matter how challenging or difficult your situation.

iRest was developed by Dr. Richard Miller, a spiritual teacher, author, yogic scholar, researcher and clinical psychologist, who combined traditional yogic practice with western psychology and neuroscience. It is practiced and taught by thousands of people worldwide in a wide range of settings, including health centers, schools, community centers, yoga studios, correctional facilities and military hospitals. You can visit iRest.org to learn more.

Ultimately, anything that leads you to strong consciousness - be it through, meditation, self-reflection and quieting of the mind - is beneficial.

The ability to be in a consistent state of relaxation and peace is so crucial to sleep. A few ways you can reduce stress is by moving to a calm nurturing environment, surrendering to relaxation or engaging in more peaceful activities. These can all help turn off the fight/flight response. However, in order to reduce stress, one must value sleep, understand its importance and commit to making it a priority for their health.

Committing to consistent relaxation not only helps your sleep but also helps manage your frustration when your baby is not sleeping, thus making it more likely that you can respond rather than react. This is an important issue. The frustration you feel at your child's sleeplessness is obviously not helpful and can contribute to making it worse.

This means learning how to adjust our energetic and emotional states. Some of us might have intense energy while others are calmer. Some of us hold onto frustration while others are able to let their frustration go. How do our energetic and emotional states influence one another? What adjustments need to be made to support or co-regulate these states, especially when it comes to crying?

If you can't manage emotions like frustration, you will carry them with you everywhere you go. Why should your child suffer because your boss has just aggravated you or because your child is struggling with sleep? If you have no or little emotional control, you'll be carrying work stressors and aggravation home with you, influencing the entire household, including your newborn.

Yes, I know your baby isn't likely to be watching Netflix (at least intentionally), but the more conscious you become, the more aware you will be of the factors (noise, light, emotional distress, physical discomfort, etc.) that keep you and your baby awake. This is one of the reasons why a baby may feel his or her parent's presence overstimulating. Interestingly, the common response from mainstream sleep consultants is to remove a parent's presence from their child so their child will not be overstimulated. The rooted issue and most optimal response would be to have parents work on regulating their emotions in order to be emotionally available so that their child is not overstimulated by their presence.

Research also supports the importance of emotional availability when it comes to the quality of child sleep.

According to the article, "Bidirectional Associations between Bedtime Parenting and Infant Sleep: Parenting Quality, Parenting Practices, and their Interaction" by Lauren E. Philbrook and Douglas M. Teti in the United States National Library of Medicine,

> *A recent cross-sectional study found that more emotionally available parenting at bedtime predicted fewer mother-reported infant night wakings (Teti et al., 2010). Parental sensitivity at bedtime in particular may be critical for helping infants prepare for nighttime sleep. Because infants are tired at bedtime, they may require more parental assistance in regulating their arousal and emotions. Furthermore, as argued by Teti et al. (2010), falling asleep requires trust in the safety of the environment. Thus, by using comforting and soothing bedtime routines, mothers may promote better nighttime sleep.*

According to the article, "Maternal emotional availability at bedtime predicts infant sleep quality" by Teti DM, Kim

BR, Mayer G and Countermine in the United States
National Library of Medicine,

*In the present study, linkages were examined
between parental behaviors (maternal practices)
at bedtime, emotional availability of mothering at
bedtime, and infant sleep quality in a cross-
sectional sample of families with infants between 1
and 24 months of age. Observations of maternal
behaviors and maternal emotional availability
were conducted independently by 2 sets of trained
observers who were blind to data being coded by
the other. With infant age statistically controlled,
specific maternal behaviors at bedtime were
unrelated to infant sleep disruptions at bedtime
and during the night. By contrast, emotional
availability of mothering at bedtime was
significantly and inversely related to infant sleep
disruption, and, although these links were
stronger for younger infants, they were significant
for older infants as well. Maternal emotional
availability was also inversely linked with
mothers' ratings of whether their infants had sleep
difficulties. These findings demonstrate that*

parents' emotional availability at bedtimes may be as important, if not more important, than bedtime practices in predicting infant sleep quality. Results support the theoretical premise that parents' emotional availability to children in sleep contexts promotes feelings of safety and security and, as a result, better-regulated child sleep.

The environment we sleep in is crucial. We form associations with our environment in many different ways - often without being aware of it. As a result. creating a sleep sanctuary is important. Think spa-like energy. If you want your child to feel peaceful and loved in this sanctuary, then it is not a place to get mad, or yell, or display anger and frustration. It is a place of ease, relaxation, safety, comfort and love.

In many cases, I have worked with well-informed and thoughtful parents who underestimate the importance of consistency and a regular routine - not only in their child's life - but in their own as well. Regular transitional routines that signal the beginning of the sleep cycle are also key to supporting your baby's sleep development.

Sleep Timing & Schedule

It seems like almost every sleep expert, regardless of his or her approach, recommends getting children on a regular sleeping schedule. Adults, like children, also benefit from being on a regular sleeping schedule. A regular, consistent and somewhat flexible schedule is key.

While there will be different sleep requirements and sleep and wake window lengths for different ages and stages, within the same age and stage, schedules and sleep requirements can greatly vary.

The National Sleep Foundation recommends that a newborn (0-3 months) sleeps a total of 14-17 hours within a 24-hour period. However, according to their requirements, anywhere from 11-13 hours of sleep or a total of 18-19 hours' sleep may also be appropriate.

If you research wake windows for a newborn, you'll find that some will say 1-2 hours of a wake window is appropriate, some will say 60-90 minutes, and some will say 45-75 minutes.

With such varying sleep requirements, how does one know the appropriate wake window length and total numbers of hours of sleep in a 24-hour period required for their newborn?

Some parents just listen to the advice and estimated number given to them by their doctor or sleep consultant and enforce it upon their child without observing and learning about their child's body cues, natural clock, rhythm and flow. As a result, they may become frustrated and stressed when their child's sleep does not fit into the advised number.

Other parents don't go by any schedule. They just go with the flow without knowing the range of total sleep requirements and wake window length, but because they are not familiar with the internal or external influences of sleep or how it works, they may also find themselves frustrated and stressed when their child is overtired or not sleeping well.

There are many factors that can affect our sleep timing and schedule. Some of these factors include:

- Light/Dark cycles
- Emotions

- Nutrition
- Circadian rhythm disruptions
- Sleep consolidation or lack of
- The range of 24-hour sleep totals
- The exact night total which will result in different wake windows and nap totals
- Sleep quality
- Sleep deficits
- Activity level
- Lifestyle
- The balance of activity and rest throughout the day

In the same way Sadhguru suggests we learn to read our user's manual; we also must also learn to read our children's user's manual.

According to psychology professor Robert Epstein, in his article "What Makes a Good Parent?" in Scientific American's magazine edition of *Secrets of Successful Parenting*, Amazon offers more than 180,000 parenting guides—more than double the number of diet books.

With so many guides available, one would assume parenting challenges are on the decline. Despite the many supportive and insightful guides to parenting and child sleep, an overwhelming number of parents still struggle.

One of the reasons parents continue to struggle is due to their sole reliance on external sources to obtain knowledge for how their body, their child's body and family dynamics function best.

Obtaining knowledge and learning from external sources is very helpful and needed. But we also must learn to develop a keen sense of awareness and rely on the intelligence of our own body. If you take the time to slow down, observe and listen, you will find the many ways your body and your child's body are communicating with you. When you begin to observe yourself and your child while remaining open, you will strengthen your consciousness and learn so much that will make it clear which sleep requirements are most optimal.

Sometimes what our child has a hard time with, we do as well. For example, challenges that have arisen with our child's sleep timing and schedule may just in fact reflect imbalances in own sleep schedule. If our lives are disorganized or inconsistent, our children may also reflect these qualities and provide us an opportunity to get organized and structured in such a way that is not only beneficial for them but for ourselves.

The Relationship Between Sleep and Emotion

Another overlooked but incredibly important area in sleep is emotional health. Unresolved or suppressed emotions can especially influence our sleep. Uncovering and processing them will not only lead to improving sleep but overall well-being.

In Grant Hilary Brenner, MD's article "How Suppressed Emotions Enter Our Dreams and Affect Health", he writes:

> *Can we "get rid" of thoughts? What happens when we believe we are throwing away mental garbage? It's one thing to stop ourselves from engaging in futile masochism or interrupt obsessive thoughts. It's another thing entirely to try to ignore important parts of oneself, joyful or melancholy. Like the global ecosystem, the ecology of the psyche dictates that we can't quite get rid of things. We push feelings into unconsciousness, but they remain implicit, having impact on our unconscious waking process and emerging in the evening. We can suppress, medicate and ignore our dreams, but when we do so we may be risking missing out on ultimately*

necessary and catalytic experiences required at times for personal development.

You can run, but you can't hide.
Prior research (Malinowski 2015) has confirmed the relevance of "dream rebound". When we suppress waking thoughts, they show up in our dreams. A recent study builds on that prior work to look at whether there is a difference in dream rebound for suppressors of positive versus negative emotions, whether this affects sleep quality, and relates to experiencing depression, anxiety or stress.

Participants who suppressed thoughts expressed within dreams more negative thoughts from waking life compared with lower suppressors. They endorsed greater levels of sadness, anger, fear and anxiety.

In addition, people with higher degrees of thought suppression and thought intrusion had poorer sleep quality as evidenced by subjective report, difficulty falling asleep, sleep disturbance, use of

sleep medication, and daytime tiredness. Those
with greater tendencies toward thought
suppression and thought intrusion had higher
levels of depression, anxiety and stress.

When it comes to infant and young children, we may
typically assume they respond to what is going on
internally, but tend to believe that external events are
beyond their understanding, and therefore their feelings.
However, it is a grave mistake to think that just because
babies and infants can't fully understand what is going on
in their environment, they are immune to it.

The fact is that babies and infants, in fact children of all
ages, feel. They may experience different levels of
sensitivity to their internal and external environment and
circumstances, but the point is that they are having an
experience. If their experience is negative, traumatic or
left unresolved, it can affect not only their development
but their ability to sleep well.

This sensitivity is even present in the womb. There,
babies start attaching to the mother through the sound of
her voice. They learn the rhythm of their native language,
an important variable in the practical use of speech. In the

womb, babies can experience the effects of mother's smoking, alcohol and medication use, as well as her moods and stresses. They are already connected to the world through the mother's experiences and her responses to them. Some have argued that the fetus can also sense fear, ambivalence, and even respond to her well-being or lack thereof.

The film In Utero, released in October 2016, is a documentary about life in the womb and its lasting impact on human development, human behavior, and the state of the world. It's become clear that the film has opened doors to some of the more critical issues of our time: how in utero development profoundly affects the rest of our lives and, as a consequence, the health of humanity.

"How we begin is who we become," In Utero's tagline states.

And then there is the birth itself. Procedures like C-sections and medications for the mother can also impact this incredible transformation. For example, the use of exogenous oxytocin (Syntocinon/Pitocin) has drawn concerns that this drug designed to facilitate labor actually reaches the fetus. This could potentially change oxytocin receptors in the brain of the fetus, which could influence the child's ability to relate to others thus impacting lifetime feelings of love and connection.

Then there are babies who are in the wrong position for birth. They are often pushed and pulled with forceps that can in some cases lead to head or neck injuries. Some children struggle long after birth with the painful effects of these procedures, affecting their sleep immediately.

Early traumas can set the child up for a lifetime of anxiety, dysfunction and addiction. These events wire the brain in a particular way, setting up defensive or dysfunctional behaviors that might last a lifetime.

While it is quite possible that such wiring does occur, we should also remember that a child's brain is constantly changing through learning. These traumas don't necessarily have to have lifelong effects. As long as there is the opportunity for the child to develop adaptive responses through loving connections and many healing therapies, these traumas can be transformed into opportunities for resilience and human expansion.

The connection between the infant and its parents and other family members is crucial in providing security from which the baby can grow and develop in a healthy way.

Dr. Gabor Maté, is a Hungarian-born Canadian physician with a background in family practice and a special interest in childhood development and trauma, potential lifelong impacts of trauma on physical and mental health, including on autoimmune disease, cancer, ADHD, addictions and a wide range of other conditions.

He says, "If you're stressed so is your kid. The more stressed parents are, the more developmental problems you will find in kids. The electrical circuitry of a child's brain is programmed by the mother's emotional state." He also says the key to raising healthy children is a nurturing home and community, but that those environments are extinct.

In many ways, sleep is both an indicator of these issues and an opportunity to find the proper treatment for them. A child having difficulty sleeping may be reflecting trauma and distress, which is why I consider a child sleep issue a family issue and why a complete environmental and family assessment is necessary. A child in a tense environment will reflect that tension in his or her body, and that will almost always disrupt quality sleep.

I'll never forget the day one of my professionals contacted me and thanked me for highlighting the connection between trauma and sleep in my Maternity and Child Sleep Certification program. She had been working with a client whose one-and-a-half-year-old child was waking up between ten and twelve times at night. After working on many sleep factors and establishing healthy sleep foundations, she helped her client's child reduce nightly wake-ups to five times per night. While this was a huge improvement, the sleep consultant continued to dig deeper into the situation. As a result, she learned that since her client had had her baby, feelings of anxiety and fear resurfaced from a memory of an abusive experience she had when she was six years old. However, since her child was so young, and mom kept her feelings hidden, it did not cross her mind that her unresolved childhood experience could be influencing her own child's sleep. The sleep consultant recommended and referred her client to therapist who could support her. After the first session, her baby slept through the night.

Sleep also serves an important function on emotional development and intelligence. Recent research sheds some very interesting light on the function of sleep and helps explain its role in the consolidation of memories and emotional processing.

The research suggests that during REM (rapid eye movement) dream sleep, emotional events are processed. During this phase of sleep, the autonomic nervous system (which underpins the stress response) is turned off. This suggests that the processing of emotions can occur without the accompanying stress reaction. In other words, REM sleep is an opportunity to process and potentially defuse emotional events leading to greater emotional intelligence and adaptation.

Additionally, there is evidence that during deeper, SWS -- slow wave sleep -- emotional memories are paired with similar but less stressful memories, thus putting them in context and defusing them of their emotion.

These findings have enormous implications for child sleep.

First, the evidence of the role of both REM and SWS in defusing emotional memories is much stronger in children than in adults. Remember, children are trying to make sense of the world and seeking security. It makes sense therefore, that childhood and even infants' sleep is very critical for their sense of security and the development of their emotional control.

Second, babies experience a lot more REM than older children and adults. Could it be that their REM and SWS are critical parts of their adaptation and thus their development?

When we don't have a good night's sleep as adults, we often feel cranky and irritable the following day. We put it down to just being tired and having less energy. However, maybe we are more stressed and emotional the following day because we haven't got into REM and as a result, our fight/flight system hasn't had a chance to turn off, allowing the moderation of our emotional state and memories.

According to the Anxiety and Depression Association of America, about 7% of Americans have a social anxiety disorder.

In one of their articles "Social Anxiety Disorder and Alcohol Abuse", the author writes, "About 20 percent of people with social anxiety disorder also suffer from alcohol abuse or dependence, and a recent study found that the two disorders have a stronger connection among women."

The common assumption is that people who have some sort of anxiety are prone to drink alcohol to manage it. However, drinking like this makes them more likely to be dependent, which leads to tolerance, which leads to more drinking and an increase in the severity of that dependency. As a result, this pattern of drinking leads to more anxiety, and the vicious cycle continues.

However, there is another possible explanation for this merry-go-round.

If you have ever worked in an alcohol rehabilitation facility, one of the most notable and consistent patterns of behavior during rehab is that after about three weeks of detox, patients suddenly report the return of dreams, very vivid dreams. This phenomenon is called REM Rebound. Regular and fairly heavy alcohol intake significantly reduces, and even eliminates the REM stage of sleep and dreaming. Heavy drinkers can go for years without any REM sleep.

If REM sleep is critical to the process of emotional management and control, going without REM will have major implications in that it will amp up emotions, which might increase your chances of drinking and suppressing REM. There's a vicious cycle here. Imagine someone with PTSD, who needs this emotional consolidation of memory perhaps more than anyone else, drinking heavily and thus not giving themselves a chance at effective emotional processing.

Of course, it's not just alcohol that can suppress the REM stage of sleep. As mentioned in the section of the impact of lifestyle on sleep, certain foods can also curtail sleep and impact REM. And that would make you crankier and less emotionally capable the following day. Not a good state for a parent to be in.

Similarly, if your infant is not getting the REM she needs, she might also be crankier. She might be crankier not just because she has less energy, but crankier because she is not adapting too well to the ups and downs of life.

Unless they are living in traumatic circumstances, aren't most children naturally stable and balanced? No, and here's why.

Layers of Connection

It is very easy to underestimate an infant or child's need for love, connection and security. There are several reasons why it is easy to overlook a child's needs.

First, in western culture, there is an excessive emphasis on independence. The notion is reified and held as the measure of health and success. However, nature, including human nature, is just as much about interdependence.

In Bonnie Ware's book, *The Five Regrets of the Dying,* many of those near the end of their lives regretted not investing more in their relationships. We say, but often pay lip service to, the notion that relationships are the key part of our lives. We have minimized the impact of our social environments.

This shows up in the child sleep industry where there is often a lot of emphasis, expectation and pressure on independent sleep and function. In addition, there is much fear that if a child cannot learn how to self-soothe and sleep on their own even as young as six months, it is a problem.

Second, we can easily underestimate the impact of the social environment on infants and even children. We often fail to see the world from their perspective.

One of my favorite stories of this phenomenon concerns a case study that was presented about a young boy of about five.

One night, the young boy started to have horrendous nightmares completely out of the blue. They began to dominate his waking as well as his sleeping moments. He imagined that there were all sorts of monsters lurking in the walls of his bedroom, and they were out to get him.

His parents became so worried about his delusions that they put him into psychotherapy, where he stayed for a year. He wasn't getting any better until one day, someone worked out what had happened.

Just prior to his breakdown, the air conditioning in the family home started to fail. A contractor was brought in to assess the situation. And the young boy overheard the contractor tell his parents, in a very serious and concerned fashion, that "there are very bad ducts in the boy's room." Except the boy heard it as, "there are very bad ducks in the boy's room." No delusion, no neurosis, just a young child misunderstanding an adult conversation.

Children are designed to be aware and sensitive to their environments. They are learning about them. When a baby comes to life on earth, he knows the sound of his mother's voice, but not much else. Your baby girl may look calm and relaxed, but typically that is because at that moment, she feels safe. Safe with her parent(s), safe in the environment, safe in all the sensory information she is receiving. However, she is also sensitive, ultra-sensitive, because she needs to be.

The cultural independence imperative often clashes with the child's sensitivity and need to adapt and learn. Babies and children have an immense need for secure attachment, bonding and connection. Secure attachment is critical. Without it, a child will feel anxious at the very least. This is true for anyone even an adult. Imagine flying to a foreign country where you know absolutely no one and nothing about the culture. You are left alone to find your way amongst strangers who don't even talk like you or look like you. Feeling defensive and anxious? You bet.

This raises the issue of what is meant by "independence" in the context of child behavior and infant sleep. Independent behavior from a baby or child means that they can do something on their own, but it doesn't mean that they are not influenced and dependent on their social environment and key relationships. A toddler who can walk on her own is doing that behavior independently, but is still very dependent on her social environment. Independent behavior is not a sign of independence in a general sense. Ironically, the more emotionally secure in their interdependence, the more likely that children will feel more comfortable acting without help, like sleeping on their own. Insisting on a child's independence without them having security and comfort in their interdependence, is illogical and counterproductive.

There are all sorts of things that can make a child feel insecure. Tension between family members at home will change the atmosphere and potentially scare a child or even an infant, even if they can't articulate that.

Unpredictable behavior from anyone in the household can upset everyone's routine and sense of security. If there's one thing that humans desperately want, it's a sense of security, a sense of control. That might manifest differently at various life stages, but the principle is surely there at every stage of life.

The moods of family members and the energy in the room will also be communicated to infants. They may not understand the subtleties of moods or be able to articulate them, but that doesn't mean they are not affected by them.

Changes in routine can also be unsettling for an infant. With any situation that can create tension, the better bonded the child is with the family, the more secure the child will feel. Security will create adaptability and resilience - exactly what is needed for learning.

Obsession with focusing on a specific behavior, like sleeping, can result in the big picture and context in which the behavior occurs to be lost. Behaviors cannot be taken out of context. When they are, they are likely to be misunderstood, misdiagnosed and not effectively managed.

The notion of attachment was expressed as Attachment Theory by John Bowlby and researched significantly by Mary Ainsworth in various settings. They proposed four types of attachment of differing degrees:

Secure attachment describes a situation in which a child is distressed on the departure of their caregiver but can reassure themselves and regain composure because they trust that the caregiver will return.

Ambivalent attachment describes children who become distressed at the departure of their caregiver and cannot reassure or soothe themselves. This implies a lack of trust and by implication, safety.

Avoidant attachment describes children who avoid their caregiver and aren't distressed when they leave. Their reactions to the caregiver are similar to their reactions to strangers. Obviously, this suggests a seriously impaired relationship.

Disoriented attachment describes children who seem to have no consistent way to manage their attachments.

Trust, safety and emotional self-management are important factors in these various attachment styles.

It's highly likely that these attachment styles influence the development of relationships and social interactions, but not to the exclusion of other variables, like relationships with other children. Nonetheless, it's generally understood that secure attachment in infancy is associated with better life adjustment.

References

Ainsworth MD, Blehar M, Waters E, Wall S (1978). Patterns of Attachment: A Psychological Study of the

Strange Situation. Hillsdale NJ: Lawrence Erlbaum Associates.

Bowlby J (1988). A Secure Base: Clinical Applications of Attachment Theory. London: Routledge.

Bowlby J (1995) [1950]. Maternal Care and Mental Health. The master work series (2nd ed.). Northvale, NJ; London: Jason Aronson. ISBN 1-56821-757-9. OCLC 33105354. [Geneva, World Health Organization, Monograph series no. 3]

A child of any age will be impacted by rapidly changing events, any sign of trouble or stress in their internal and external worlds or anything that's new or different. If these traumas and stresses are not relieved and managed, there's a chance that they will indeed evolve into long-term challenges.

An infant manages his world through seeking secure attachment with his or her relationship with a parental figure, typically mother. In some cases, that parental figure is dad, or a surrogate mother figure or even a grandparent. Without such a secure and constant attachment, that child will be constantly off-balance, stressed and likely to develop maladaptive behaviors that can turn into lifelong tragedies.

A secure attachment allows the child to develop confidence in themselves and others. They feel sure of the support and love that is implicit in that secure attachment. There is nothing as beautiful as a loving, nurturing connection - nor as important.

Attachment Theory has spawned research that has confirmed that although all parent-caregiver child relationships are important, the mother-child relationship is considered a critical variable in infant development. It forms the core of the child's ability to cope, manage relationships and even the development of personality. When the biological mother is absent from a child's world, the child can form a similar attachment with another parent-caregiver supporting the child's development.

Behaviorally, attachment protects the child and helps her in safely navigating the world. Such behaviors include clinging, sucking, and movement - all of which contribute to physical, emotional and neurological development. In short, babies rely on their primary caregivers to lovingly guide them through the world, helping them to develop adaptive behaviors in the process.

This secure attachment also comes into play with sleep. However, the mother or father choose to manage infant sleep, it should always be done with love and the conveyed assurance that the baby will remain safe and secure.

The attachment between mother and child is an evolving, interdependent relationship. Research shows that mothers who are attuned to their child's physical and emotional states, create and reinforce their relationship.

A definition of attunement 'is a kinesthetic and emotional sensing of others knowing their rhythm, affect and experience by metaphorically being in their skin, and going beyond empathy to create a two-person experience of unbroken feeling connectedness by providing a reciprocal affect and/or resonating response'. (Erksine 1998)

Attunement means the mother attends to, and understands, her baby's signals and this will lead to satisfaction for both parties. If a mother's attunement is off, or doesn't exist, then it may lead to distress in both the baby and the mother.

Susan Stearn, LCSW and founder of The Social Skills Place writes:

> *Attunement has a lot to do with our abilities in non-verbal communication. In fact, most of our communication with our children and others is non-verbal and a large percentage of what our brains perceive in communication with others is non-verbal signals. Some examples of our day-to-day signals to our children or others may be the movement of your eye (a warm wink), facial gestures, (the opening of your mouth in surprise, a yawn) your tone of voice, the movement of your hand (a wave, or an A-OK) or the tip of your head. And most of the time we are unaware of any of our non-verbal gestures. We just do them. We even repeat our own parent's non-verbal gestures to us. It is important to know your child can*

literally sense your interest and sincerity in them,
as well your approval or disapproval in them.
Attunement and attachment are related.

In order to have the ability to attune to another, we must be attuned to ourselves. A challenge I have come across with many clients and professionals in not only in the sleep industry, but in general is that attunement often is overshadowed by reliance on external sources via books, articles and controversial advice given by experts.

There is also such an overload of information that it is very easy for one to get lost in it and forget the inner guidance that contains valuable intelligence and information.

While outside information can be helpful, solely relying on it without attuning to oneself prevents us from fully understanding ourselves and one another. It also prevents us from fully connecting to the challenges we or our children are facing in order to find the right solution.

Lastly, I have found play and gratitude are often missing pieces with families experiencing child sleep challenges.

They both can offer a tremendous opportunity to overcome challenges pretty quickly.

Play

"Life is too important to be taken seriously." ~ Oscar Wilde

How often do you play with your child or on your own?

Many of us have forgotten how to play and have fun, especially with our children. Play brings joy and joy is a necessary emotion for our state of well-being. Play allows us to connect, feel safe, relax and heal, which are all necessary for optimal sleep. Play is critical for problem solving, creativity, and relationships.

Dr. Bowen White, physician and founding member of the National Institute for Play, says *"Play is essential to our health. It's a way of life that allows you to let your guard down, not be so serious and, as a result, connect better with others. It has the opposite effect on the body as stress. Play often leads to laughter, which has been linked to decreased stress and inflammation and may improve vascular health."

Dr. Stuart Brown, founder of the National Institute for Play, says there is a strong connection between the practice of play and the emotional and cognitive development of the brain. Even simply giggling with your child will improve their physical and emotional well-being.

When physical and emotional well-being are improved, sleep is improved.

Gratitude

For most people, feeling gratitude when faced with a challenge seems almost impossible. However, cultivating gratitude on a regular basis helps us manage stress more effectively, connect easier with others, strengthens our immune system, lowers blood pressure and improves our overall state of well-being.

According to a white paper prepared for the John Templeton Foundation by the Greater Good Science

Center at UC Berkeley by Summer Allen, Ph.D., on The
Science of Gratitude,

*A handful of studies suggest that more grateful
people may be healthier, and others suggest that
scientifically designed practices to increase
gratitude can also improve people's health and
encourage them to adopt healthier habits. Many
more studies have examined possible
connections between gratitude and various
elements of psychological well-being. In general,
more grateful people are happier, more satisfied
with their lives, less materialistic, and less likely
to suffer from burnout. Additionally, some
studies have found that gratitude practices, like
keeping a "gratitude journal" or writing a letter
of gratitude, can increase people's happiness and
overall positive mood. Gratitude may also benefit
people with various medical and psychological
challenges. For example, one study found that
more grateful cardiac patients reported better
sleep, less fatigue, and lower levels of cellular
inflammation, and another found that heart
failure patients who kept a gratitude journal for*

eight weeks were more grateful and had reduced signs of inflammation afterwards. Several studies have found that more grateful people experience less depression and are more resilient following traumatic events.

The Illusion of Quick Fixes and Guarantees

Adopt the pace of nature: her secret is patience.
~ Ralph Waldo Emerson

If I were to ask most health, lifestyle and sleep coaches what they feel pressured by the most when working with clients, many will share they feel pressured to provide their clients quick solutions and results.

We live in a society that thrives on short cuts and instant fixes. As a result, we forget that many solutions and goals require time.

While instant fixes can happen and have their place from time to time, the reality is that many solutions require time in order to obtain long term results. Many challenges we experience are due to health and lifestyle habits that took a while to condition and will take a while to reshape.

When we demand or feel pressured to have quick results, we usually go to extremes to accomplish them, thus experiencing short term outcomes. As a result, full evaluations, gradual transitions and progress leading to long term results are often are overlooked and not given the value they deserve.

If a potential client approaches me and wants me to ensure her that I will provide her quick results, I let her know up front that my approach is holistic and whether a result is quick or will take time depends on many factors.

"Success is a journey, not a destination. The doing is often more important than the outcome." ~ Arthur Ashe

It is very easy to lose sight of the progress you have made if you are focused on the end goal rather than the journey. And because of this, it is also easier to remain frustrated when your end goal has not happened, so you find yourself becoming negative or discouraged.

Another issue I see often is coaches and consultants offering guaranteed results. If I am being honest with myself and with my clients, I cannot guarantee someone else's actions or behavior. My clients are responsible and accountable for that. While one can attempt to do their best to control or enforce another's behavior, as I wrote earlier, enforcing behavior can lead to resistance and negative behaviors.

What I can guarantee is my support, guidance and shining the light on areas my clients are in the dark about. I can guarantee my commitment to a collaborative process where we work together as team. I can guarantee a thorough investigative process that gets to the root of my clients' sleep challenges. I can also guarantee my knowledge, experience, professionalism, timeliness, attention.

But to guarantee that my client or their child will resolve their sleep challenges in a few days is very misleading.

We also have become accustomed to expecting immediate

It is up to us to take full responsibility for our choices and quality of life. In doing so, we empower ourselves to be more receptive, naturally driven and motivated to seek, reflect and connect with our inner guide. When we begin to develop a stronger connection and relationship with our body, we will be guided to take the appropriate solution-oriented actions for ourselves and our children and that may require adopting nature's pace.

Finding Solutions

If you have consulted with your doctor but still have trouble sleeping, you are not alone. It is also not uncommon for me to work with clients, who after seeing their doctor or therapist for help with sleep challenges, still continue to experience them. This is primarily because there are many health and lifestyle factors that are not thoroughly being investigated or effectively being addressed to uncover the root cause of a sleep challenge.

In order to understand why, let's first consider the background, training and experience of doctors when it comes to sleep. Did you know, for example, that doctors, including pediatricians, only receive two to four hours total of general sleep education in medical school? Most general doctors, unless educated holistically, are trained to treat the symptoms and not the cause. In addition, they generally do not have time to spend going into such depth with their clients to support sleep education, prevention, perform a thorough investigation, advise or manage a patient's health and lifestyle behaviors.

For example, according to a BMC, published study, "Sleep education in pediatric residency programs: a cross-cultural look"- Overall, the average amount of time spent on sleep education is 4.4 hours (median = 2.0 hours), with 23% responding that their pediatric residency program provides no sleep education. Almost all programs (94.8%) offer less than 10 hours of instruction. The predominant topics covered include sleep-related development, as well as normal sleep, sleep-related breathing disorders, parasomnias, and behavioral insomnia of childhood.

.

According to Harvard Medical School, "The most recent survey of the four-year medical school curriculum reveals an average of less than two hours of formal education directed at sleep, even at Harvard Medical School."

.

In 2011 Dr. Daniel Goh at the National University Children's Medical Institute in Singapore sent surveys to 409 medical schools in 12 countries to see how they compared in their sleep curriculum. The appalling results show the U.S., along with Australia, ahead of the pack, with around three hours spent on the subject of sleep-in classrooms or in residency. Indonesia, Malaysia and Vietnam reported zero hours.

.

Before taking sleep advice from your primary doctor for your child or for yourself, find out how much sleep education and experience they have and whether they have undergone additional training to support their sleep education.

Next, let's take a look at sleep doctors "somnologists", also referred to as sleep specialists and the important role they play in helping you find sleep solutions.

What is a sleep doctor?

According to Healthline, "A sleep specialist is a doctor who diagnoses and treats sleep disorders. Most sleep specialists train in internal medicine, psychiatry, pediatrics, or neurology during residency. After completing residency, they complete a fellowship program in sleep medicine.

Doctors who receive training in sleep medicine get their board certification from the American Board of Sleep Medicine, which is part of the American Board of Medical Specialties."

There are a variety of sleep doctors who have a special area of expertise. According to Healthline, the list includes:

- psychiatrists and psychologists, who treat thoughts and behaviors related to sleep
- neurologists, who treat brain and nervous system disorders
- pediatricians, who treat sleep disorders in children
- otorhinolaryngologists, who treat problems with the ear, nose, and throat that contribute to sleep disorders
- dentists and oral and maxillofacial surgeons, who fit people for oral appliances to correct problems with the mouth and jaw
- respiratory therapists, who work with sleep doctors to manage and treat breathing disorders

The conditions sleep specialists most often treat include:

- Insomnia
- Sleep apnea
- Narcolepsy
- Restless leg syndrome

- Circadian rhythm disorders
- Parasomnia

While sleep doctors have successfully helped many of their patients, many others continue to struggle. There can be many reasons for this, but a primary reason is that sleep doctors do not provide accountability for health and lifestyle habits and behavior changes necessary for their patients to sustain a long-term solution. Sleep doctors also place their primary focus on the diagnosis of sleep disorders and the treatments versus performing a thorough investigation leading to uncover the root cause of their patient's sleep challenge.

This is where sleep coaches come in.

What is a sleep coach?

According to the Boston's Children Hospital, "A sleep coach, or sleep consultant, is a general term for someone who provides education, advice and support services to help improve sleep. However, the criteria for who can call themselves a "sleep coach" can be quite variable and the term does not guarantee any specific training or certification. So, when choosing a sleep coach, be sure to do your homework about the coach's background, training and previous experience to determine if he or she is the right fit for you."

In the United States, for example, coaching isn't regulated by any state or federal agency. There is no licensing requirement for the sleep coaching profession like there is for medical doctors or therapists. And with the increase in demand for sleep support, more pop-up certification programs from sleep coaches, with different philosophies, who may have a background in sleep, but not in curriculum development or professional training, are popping up. Just because you are a successful sleep coach does not automatically make you a great teacher who's qualified to teach professionals about sleep. To be a great teacher, the following skills are required:

- An understanding of different learning styles and approaches
- Works effectively in groups
- Is able to deal with conflict neutrally and non-judgmentally
- Motivates and empowers students to do their best

- Encourages questioning and ideas from students
- Practices patience and empathy with students
- Shares constructive and empowering feedback to students
- An avid researcher
- Continuously provides updates to the course curriculum
- Actively listens to students
- Collaborates with other colleagues
- Role models leadership
- Knows how to explain digestible content and demonstrate practical application
- Incorporates class surveys and maintains open communication
- Is forward thinking

What qualifies a sleep coach?

To ensure you are working with a highly qualified sleep coach professional who is adhering to the finest standards and best practices, ask how many hours of training both in theory and practice they have had, what kind of approach they follow and how they conduct their sessions.

A qualified sleep coach is professionally trained and certified in sleep science, health and education and learns the skills of:

- Signs and symptoms of medical conditions to know when and how to refer out
- active listening
- powerful questioning, such as motivational interviewing
- tracking progress and accountability
- practical and realistic planning and goal setting
- establishing a coaching presence
- categorizing and prioritizing short term and long-term goals
- performing a thorough investigation and evaluation
- uncovering the root cause of their client's challenge

Their training involves both theory and practice and at least a minimum of one hundred hours of education, including being mentored through case studies and working with volunteers. Qualified sleep coaches are also required to maintain their education by renewing their credentials usually every two years with proof of continued education and do not diagnose, examine or treat their clients.

In addition, qualified sleep coaches also learn how to be in a collaborative relationship with their clients in order to provide their clients an opportunity to learn about themselves, increase their self-worth and control the decision-making process. Doing so motivates clients to carry out actions that are of interest and value to them leading to behavioral change that initiated from self-autonomy and not from dependency on their sleep coach. Essentially, they become your personal cheerleader, guide and partner empowering you to take charge of your sleep health.

The best solution seems for sleep doctors and sleep coaches to work together. The good news is that, this is now happening.

Health coaches, which includes sleep coaches, are now being recognized by the medical industry as playing a vital role to assist with prevention, management and accountability of the health and lifestyle behaviors of their patients.

According to the American Medical Association:
.

"Having a health coach involved in a patient's care can not only increase patient satisfaction and engagement but also reduce physician stress and burnout by freeing up time. A health coach can bring an extra boost to your practice's methods for both prevention and treatment."

According to the Institute for Functional Medicine:

"Working alongside a clinician, health coaches advise and motivate patients to change unhealthy lifestyle habits and manage chronic conditions by providing them with tools and support to navigate when times get rough."

According to a New York Times article, "We Could All Use a Health Coach" by Jane E Brody:

"Health coaches support doctors whose time with each patient is likely to be limited to 12 to 15 minutes.

"The doctor may tell a patient 'Eat less, exercise more, take your medicine and come back in three months,' but not how to execute this plan," said Dr. Rushika Fernandopulle, a primary care doctor in Hyannis, Mass.

As founder of Iora Health, a national network of primary care practices, Dr. Fernandopulle has made health coaches an integral part of patient care at dozens of medical sites around the country. Even if doctors had more time, he said, they're not taught — and few know how — to motivate patients to make changes that would improve their health."

What about a pediatric sleep consultant? Is a pediatric sleep consultant a child sleep doctor? The majority of the case, no. Unless a pediatric sleep consultant has a medical license, technically they are not considered to be pediatric. The definition of "pediatric" according to the Oxford dictionary is defined as. "relating to the branch of medicine dealing with children and their diseases." That being the case, most pediatric sleep consultants fundamentally are just sleep consultants with an inaccurate title.

Uncovering the Root Cause

There could a number of reasons for your sleep challenge. While others may be experiencing sleep challenges similar to yours, the root cause may be very different. As a result, the solution would be different and therefore, a cookie cutter or general solution that worked for someone else, may not work for you.

For example, below is an example of the various adult and pediatric sleep questionnaires sourced from the American Thoracic Society:

Adult Questionnaires

Sleep Apnea

- Sleep Disorders Questionnaire (SDQ)
- Berlin Questionnaire
- STOP BANG
- OSA50
- Self-efficacy in Sleep apnea (SEMSA)
- Calgary Sleep Apnea Quality of Life Index (SAQLI)

Sleep Quality

- Functional Outcomes of Sleep Questionnaire (FOSQ)
- Pittsburgh Sleep Quality Index (PSQI)

Restless Legs Syndrome

- International Restless Legs Scale (IRLS)
- Augmentation Severity Rating Scale (ASRS)
- Restless Legs Syndrome Quality of Life Questionnaire (RLSQoL)

Circadian Rhythm

- Morningness-Eveningness Questionnaire (MEQ)
- Munich Chronotype Questionnaire (MCTQ)
- The Sleep Timing Questionnaire (STQ)

Insomnia

- Insomnia Severity Index (ISI)

Excessive Daytime Sleepiness

- Epworth Sleepiness Scale (ESS)
- Stanford Sleepiness Scale (SSS)

Narcolepsy

- Cataplexy questionnaire

Pediatric Sleep Questionnaires

Sleep habits – Infants

- Brief Infant Sleep Questionnaire (BISQ)

Sleep habits - age > 1 year

- Children's Sleep Habits Questionnaire (CSHQ)
- Pediatric Sleep questionnaire (PSQ)
- Tayside Children's Sleep Questionnaire (TCSQ)

Daytime Sleepiness

- Pediatric Daytime Sleepiness Scale (PDSS)

- Cleveland Adolescent Sleepiness Questionnaire (CASQ)
- Epworth Sleepiness Scale for Children and Adolescents (ESS-CHAD)
- Habitual Activity Estimation Scale
- ISAAC (International Study of Asthma and Allergies in Childhood) Questionnaires

Before trying any sleep solution, start with a thorough sleep evaluation that takes into consideration your health and lifestyle, and become aware of signs or symptoms that would need to be evaluated by your doctor and/or therapist for further testing. Qualified holistic sleep coaches use standard questionnaires in addition to customizing questions according to their client's specific case and refer out when necessary. Not sure if you have a sleep condition that needs medical attention? When in doubt, get it medically checked out.

Uncovering the root cause

In order to begin uncovering the possible root cause(s) that would then lead to a customized solution perfectly designed for you, and in addition to filling out a standard sleep questionnaire intake with a qualified professional, below are some examples of questions to consider and reflect on that may not always be asked by your doctor:

How often do I experience sleep challenges each week (daily, a few days a week, weekly)?

When did my sleep challenge first begin?

What decisions or actions may have led up to my current situation?

What have I tried in the past to resolve my sleep challenge and why do I feel it has not worked?

How long do I sleep each night on average and how would I rate the quality of sleep? (1 poor quality, 10 high quality)

What is my sleep schedule like during the week and on weekends (wake up time and bed time)?

Do I eat at consistent times each day or does my eating time vary each day?

Do I wake up and go to bed at consistent times each day or do my wake up and bed times vary?

Has there been a recent change in my circumstances, health or lifestyle around the time my sleep challenges began?

On a scale of 1-10 how would I rate my overall stress levels currently (1 least stressed, 10 most stressed)?

What areas of my life below do I feel the most stressed?

- Financial
- Career
- Personal
- Marriage
- Relationships
- Mental Health
- Physical Health
- Family

- Spiritual
- Unfulfilled expectations
- Other

How is my stress level compared in the morning versus the evening?

How do I respond to stress?

Do I have a healthy outlet, tool or support system to manage my stress?

Do I have any current feelings that overwhelm me at night before going to sleep, like fear or anxiety?

If so, am I willing to seek professional support to discuss them?

Do I process my emotions during the day by journaling, engaging in a creative outlet (for example singing, dancing, playing an instrument, painting, etc.) or belonging to a positive support group?

Could there be anything in my daily diet (food, drinks, medication or supplements) that is considered anti-sleep and be inhibiting my ability to sleep?

When was my last doctor's visit and the last time I had lab work done to check for nutritional deficiencies?

What times throughout the day and evening do I eat, drink, take medication or supplements? How do I feel afterward?

When is my first exposure to sunlight on an average day, for how long am I in the sun and how much sun exposure on average am I getting on a weekly basis?

What time do I usually turn my lights off in the evening?

What is the total amount of screen time I am exposed to on a daily basis?

What time in the evening do I usually turn off screens? How do I feel after turning off screens?

Does my bedroom environment feel supportive and nurturing? If not, why not?

My Sleep Environment:

- Is it completely dark?
- Would I describe my mattress as comfortable? Is it firm or soft?
- How many windows are in my bedroom?
- Are windows in my bedroom kept mostly closed or opened?
- Do I keep an alarm clock by my bed?
- Do I sleep with an iPad or smartphone by my bed?
- Do I have scented candles, air fresheners or other fragrances in my room?
- Is there are a tv or computer in my bedroom? If so, what is the latest time in the evening I watch tv before or in bed?
- What is the noise level like in my room?
- Do my pets wake me up at night?

- Is anyone I am sharing my home with, waking me up at night?

Does my work environment feel supportive to my physical and mental health? If not, why not?

Do I engage in a physical activity on a daily basis? If so, for how long?

When was the last time I felt really good?

What activities bring me most joy?

Do I consider myself an optimist or pessimist?

On a scale of 1-10, how satisfied do I feel with myself (1 least satisfied, 10 most satisfied)?

On a scale of 1-10, how confident do I feel about overcoming my personal challenges (1 least confident, 10 most confident)?

Conclusion

So much time, energy and money has been spent desperately trying to resolve our own and our child's sleep issues. Even with all the books, strategies and advice, sleep challenges are still on the rise. We live in a society that has overgeneralized, overcomplicated and exacerbated the problem by dealing with sleep challenges superficially and as a result, not uncovering the root cause. We have been misguiding ourselves with limiting thoughts, perspectives and beliefs. Yet, all these challenges present us with the opportunity to face deeper issues, like the quality of our life, our lifestyle and relationships. The time has come for a holistic approach to guide us back to optimal well-being by empowering us to develop a keen sense of awareness, strong connection to our bodies and make healthy choices toward sleep; where we no longer accept cookie cutter and generalized solutions and invite a customized approach that addresses the specific circumstances surrounding our sleep challenge. When we are well-rested, we are at ease and we are peaceful. When we are peaceful, the quality of our life and relationships improves tremendously. As a result, our world becomes a better place. Therefore, I believe sleep is essential to our human evolution.

Acknowledgements

My children, Bella and Taj, have been my greatest teachers and inspiration. I have so much appreciation and gratitude for your profound presence in my life. To my talented editor, Shanen Ilg, who offered her tremendous support, provided my book the attention and care it deserves and went above and beyond my expectations. I feel blessed, honored and grateful for you. Mark Wood, I am so grateful for your devotion to truth, health and for sharing your intelligence and resources. Thank you to every teacher throughout my lifetime who has not only provided me with tremendous insight, but has led me back to awakening to the wisdom within me. Thank you to all the child sleep experts, doctors, researchers and scientists for your dedication and contributions. Thank you to my incredible team of instructors, students and graduates of my company, International Parenting & Health Institute, who enrolled in my program with an open curiosity, believing in me and my approach. It is because of you that my Holistic Science of Sleep Method has been shared in fifty-nine countries. This book has been a true labor of love. My hope is that it supports your work and spreads the word and mission of holistic sleep. Thank you to all my clients over the last twenty-five years who have blessed me with the opportunity not only to support their well-being but have also provided me to learn from them as well.

www.ingramcontent.com/pod-product-compliance
Lightning Source LLC
Chambersburg PA
CBHW031127090426
42738CB00008B/1001